ANTI-INFLAMMATORY DIET

THE ULTIMATE GUIDE TO HEAL THE IMMUNE SYSTEM, REDUCE INFLAMMATION AND WEIGHT LOSS WITH EASY AND HEALTHY RECIPES

By Susan Lombardi

Introduction

The anti-inflammatory diet aims at ridding the body of toxins and chemicals in most normal diets and giving the body the building blocks, and it needs to heal. Reduction of inflammation can help prevent serious health problems, including heart disease and autoimmune disorders. Research suggests that the inflammation parts an important role in many of the chronic health problems which are growing in age. The anti-inflammatory diet is full of naturally occurring, whole, healthy foods. Perhaps the most important component of an anti-inflammatory diet is fruits and vegetables. Since plant-based foods are a natural source of essential vitamins and minerals, they can provide the nutrients we need without all the calories. The best vegetables are dark leafy greens like kale or spinach, which are rich in nutrients and contain antioxidants and anti-inflammatory compounds.

For a sweet treat, eat a handful of antioxidant-rich berries, or some potassium-rich banana. Don't have to be boring on salads; with carrots, peas, onions, and more to top your greens. Dairy is not banned from an anti-inflammatory diet, but experts recommend reducing the amount of whole-fat dairy that we eat when inflammation is an issue. Dairy contains plenty of saturated fat, which may increase the risk of cholesterol and heart disease, and this may reverse the champions ' good diet. Some cheeses, like feta, are, of course, better for you than their refined counterparts and can avoid the need to completely eliminate milk. Alternatives to butter, like olive oil, can also help to reduce intake.

The anti-inflammatory diet is not only a low-carbs diet, and therefore the addition of whole-grain bread, whole-grain pasta, brown rice, and other grains into meals is allowed. However, it is best to eat only whole grains, and avoid foods made from white flour and high in sugar. One excellent source is oatmeal, such as quinoa, brown rice, and many others. These whole-grain foods contain lots of fiber, promoting healthy digestion and reducing inflammation on the whole body. Use these to make salads, grain bowls, and healthy side dishes. Seafood is an important complement to an anti-inflammatory diet. If you don't like salmon, that is a popular choice, choose a milder fish like tilapia, trout or arctic char. Many fish have high omega-3 fatty acid levels that help fight inflammation and promote heart health. At least try eating seafood twice a week, preferably rather than red meat, particularly processed meat.

In volatile conditions, the book thoroughly discussed all these food components and their functions.

Chapter 1: Inflammation

Inflammation is a crucial part of the immune system's reaction to injury and infection. It is the way the body activates the immune system for healing and restoring damaged tissue, and it protects itself against foreign invaders, such as viruses and bacteria. Wounds would fester as a physiological response without treatment, and infections may turn deadly. It can, however, become problematic if the inflammatory process goes on for a longer period of time or if the inflammatory process occurs in places where it is not necessary. Chronic inflammation has been related to certain diseases such as heart disease or stroke, and can also lead to disorders that are autoimmune such as rheumatoid arthritis and lupus. But a healthy diet and lifestyle will help keep the inflammation under control.

1.1 What is Inflammation?

Consider inflammation as the body's natural response in defending itself against damage. There are two types: acute and chronic. You are probably more familiar with the acute form that happens when you strike your knee or cut your finger. Your immune system dispatches an army of WBCs that surround and protect the body, causing noticeable redness and swelling. If you contract an illness such as flu or pneumonia, the process works similarly. In these conditions, however, inflammation is necessary— without it, injuries could become festering, and simple infections could be life-threatening.

But chronic inflammation can also present in response to other unhealthy substances in the body, such as toxins from cigarette smoke or an excess of fat cells (especially belly fat). Inflammation within the arteries helps kick off atherosclerosis— the formation of a plaque that is high in fat and cholesterol. The body considers this plaque as strange and alien, so it tries to wall away from the plaque from the blood that flows in. But if that wall splits, then the plaque breaks. The contents then combine with blood, forming a clot that blocks blood flow. These clots are responsible for the bulk of heart attacks and most strokes. A simple blood test, known as the hsCRP test, can measure C-reactive protein (CRP), which is an inflammatory marker for artery inflammation. Harvard researchers found almost 20 years ago that men with higher CRP levels— around 2 milligrams per liter (mg / L) or higher — have three times the risk of heart attack and half the risk of stroke as that in men with low or no chronic inflammation. Researchers also found that the most beneficial to people with the highest degree of arterial inflammation was aspirin, a drug that helps prevent blood clots and also dampens inflammation.

Yet several doctors do not routinely recommend the hsCRP test, because they do not feel the results will primarily impact the condition. If you're young and healthy, and you're at low risk for heart disease, there's no proof that knowing your CRP level is beneficial. If you have cardiac disease, you should already take medicines such as a cholesterol-lowering statin, which reduces the risk of heart attacks. Statins do appear to work especially well, as with aspirin, in people with arterial inflammation. One research has also found that statins decrease the risk of death in individuals with normal cholesterol levels but CRP levels of 2 mg / L or greater. So, if you are middle-aged or over and have signs of potential heart problems, such as high blood pressure level, high cholesterol level, or a family history of heart disease, knowing that you have a high level of CRP that leads you into more proactive heart safety actions. These include regular aerobic exercise, and weight loss (if necessary), and avoidance of smoking.

1.2 Types of Inflammation

There are two types of inflammation:
- Acute inflammation
- Chronic Inflammation

Acute Inflammation

Acute inflammation accompanies a knee injury, a sprained ankle, or a sore throat. It's a short-term solution with localized effects, meaning it operates at the exact location where there is a problem. As per the National Library of Medicine, the telltale signs of acute inflammation include redness, swelling, heat, and at times pain and loss of function. Blood vessels dilate in the case of acute inflammation, blood flow increases, and white blood cells surround the injured area to promote healing, Dr. Scott Walker, a family practice physician at Gunnison Valley Hospital in Utah, said. This reaction is what makes the injured area red and gets swollen.

During the process of acute inflammation, the compromised tissue releases chemicals known as cytokines. The cytokines serve as "emergency signals" that carry immune cells, hormones, and nutrients into your body to fix the issue, Walker said.

In addition, hormone-like substances known as prostaglandins produce blood clots to regenerate damaged tissue and, as part of the healing process, cause pain and fever too. The acute inflammation slowly subsides as the body heals.

Chronic Inflammation

Like acute inflammation, chronic inflammation can have long-term and whole-body consequences. Chronic inflammation is also called chronic, low-grade inflammation because it causes a constant, low-level inflammation throughout the body, as measured by a small rise in immune system markers found in blood or tissue. This form of systemic inflammation can contribute to the development of the disease, according to a review in the Johns Hopkins Health Review.

Low levels of inflammation can be caused by a perceived internal threat, even when there isn't a disease to combat or an injury to treat, and sometimes this gives signals to the immune system to answer. Because of this, white blood cells swarm but have nothing to do and nowhere to go, and they may eventually start targeting internal organs or other healthy tissues and cells, Walker said.

Scientists are researching to understand the effects of chronic inflammation on the body and the processes involved in the procedure, but it's famous for playing a role in the development of a lot of diseases.

For example, heart disease and stroke have been related to chronic inflammation. One theory suggests that when inflammatory cells stay in blood vessels for too long, they promote plaque formation. According to the (AHA), the body finds this plaque to be a foreign agent that does not belong, so it seeks to wall off the plaque from the blood flowing within the arteries. When the plaque is unstable and ruptures, it forms a clot blocking the flow of blood to the heart and brain, causing a heart attack or stroke.

Cancer is another chronic inflammation-related illness. According to the National Cancer Institute, chronic inflammation can cause damage to the DNA over time and contribute to some forms of cancer.

Chronic, low-grade inflammation often does not have signs, but doctors will check for C-reactive protein (CRP), a proxy for inflammation in the blood. High levels of CRP have been associated with an increased risk of heart disease. CRP levels can also signify an illness, or a chronic inflammatory condition, such as rheumatoid arthritis or lupus, according to the Mayo Clinic.

In addition to finding clues in the blood, a person's diet, lifestyle habits, and exposures to the environment may lead to chronic inflammation. In order to keep inflammation in check, it is necessary to maintain a healthy lifestyle.

1.3 The Pathophysiology of Inflammation

There are three sub-phases in the initial phase of inflammation: acute, sub-acute, and chronic (or proliferative). The acute phase usually lasts 1–3 days and is marked by five classical signs: heat, redness, swelling, pain, and loss of function. The subacute phase can last from 3–4 days to ~ one month, and corresponds to a required pre-repair cleaning stage. If the subacute phase is not resolved within ~1 mo, then the inflammation is said to be chronic and may last several months. The tissue can degenerate, and chronic inflammation in the locomotive system can cause tearing and fracturing. While tissue can be patched and replaced after the subacute inflammatory period during the remodeling cycle.

From a mechanistic point of view, the immediate response to tissue damage occurs in the microcirculation at the injury site. Initially, arterioles are temporarily constricted; however, chemical mediators released at the site will relax arteriolar smooth muscle within a few minutes, leading to vasodilatation and increased capillary permeability. The protein-rich fluid then exudes from the capillaries into the interstitial space. This fluid includes many of the plasma components that mediate the inflammatory response, including albumin, fibrinogen, kinins, complements, and immunoglobulins.

The sub-acute cycle is characterized by moving the phagocytic cells to the site of injury. Reacting to adhesion, molecules released from activated endothelial cells, leukocytes, platelets, and erythrocytes into damaged vessels become sticky and bind to the endothelial cell surfaces. The first cells to enter the harm site, such as neutrophils, are polymorphonuclear leukocytes. Basophils and eosinophils are more common in allergic reactions or in parasites. When inflammation progresses, the macrophages predominate, selectively attacking damaged cells or tissues. If the cause of the injury is removed, then the sub-acute phase of inflammation that follows a period of tissue repair. Fibrinolysis removes the blood clots, and fibroblasts, collagen, or endothelial cells repair or replace weakened tissues. The new collagen produced during the repair phase (mainly type III) is gradually replaced by type I collagen, in order to conform to the original tissue during the remodeling process. However, if inflammation is chronic, the tissue and/or fibrosis can deteriorate further.

1.4 Chemical Mediators of Inflammation

Biochemical mediators released during inflammation amplify and spread the inflammatory response (see the Inflammatory Mediator Actions). These mediators are soluble, diffusible molecules and can act locally and systemically. Plasma-derived mediators include complimentary, and regulated peptides and kinins. Released through the classic or alternative pathways of the supplement cascade, complement-derived peptides (C3a, C3b, and C5a) enhance vascular permeability, cause smooth muscle contraction, stimulate leukocytes, and induce mast cell degranulation. C5a is an important chemical component for neutrophils and mononuclear phagocytes. The kinins are important inflammatory mediums too. Bradykinin is the most active kinin that increases vascular permeability and vasodilation and, most importantly, promotes the release of arachidonic acid (AA) by phospholipase A2 (PLA2). Bradykinin is also a big mediator involved in the pain response. Other mediators are derived from damaged tissue or leukocyte cells, which are recruited to the site of inflammation. The serotonin and histamine vasoactive amines produce mast cells, platelets, and basophilia. Histamine induces arteriolar dilation, increased capillary permeability, smooth non-vascular muscle contraction, and eosinophilic chemotaxis, and may induce nociceptors of the pain response. The release is caused by complements from C3a and C5a, and lysosomal proteins released from neutrophils. Histamine activity is regulated by activation of one of four specific histamine receptors, called H1, H2, H3, or H4, in target cells. The majority of histamine-induced vascular effects are mediated by H1 receptors. H2 receptors mediate certain vascular effects but are more important due to their role in the histamine-caused gastric secretion. The function of H3 receptors, which may be located at the CNS, is less understood. H4 receptors are present on hematopoietic cells, and H4 antagonists are promising drug candidates for treating inflammatory conditions that involve mast cells and eosinophils (allergic conditions). Serotonin (5-hydroxytryptamine) is a vasoactive, associated histamine mediator present in the GI and CNS tracts of mast cells and platelets. Serotonin also enhances vascular permeability, dilates capillaries, and causes smooth muscle contraction, which is non-vascular. In few species, including rodents and domestic ruminants, serotonin may be the dominant vasoactive amine.

Cytokines, including IL 1–10, tumor necrosis factor α (TNF-α), and interferon γ (INF-α), are generated predominantly by macrophages and lymphocytes, but can also be synthesized by other cell types. When it comes to inflammation, their function is complex. These polypeptides modulate the actions of other cells and function towards organizing and controlling the inflammatory response. Two of the most effective cytokines, interleukin-1 (IL-1) and TNF-α, mobilize and activate leucocytes, increase the proliferation of B and T cells and increase the cytotoxicity of the natural killer cells, and are involved in the biological response to endotoxins. IL-1, IL-6, and TNF-α mediate acute phase response and pyrexia that may accompany the infection and may cause systemic clinical signs, including sleep and anorexia. In the acute phase response, interleukins enable the liver to synthesize acute-phase proteins, including the complement components, protease inhibitors, and metal-binding proteins. Cytokines are also necessary to induce PLA2 by increasing concentrations of intracellular Ca2+ in the leukocytes. Colony-stimulating factors are cytokines that promote the expansion of neutrophil, eosinophil, and macrophage colonies by the bone marrow. CytokinesIL-1, IL-6, and TNF-α contribute to the activation of fibroblasts and osteoblasts in chronic inflammation and the excretion of enzymes such as collagenase and stromelysin that can activate cartilage and bone resorption. Experimental evidence also confirms that cytokines stimulate synovial cells and chondrocytes to trigger the pain-causing mediators.

Inflammatory response, lipid-derived autacoids play a major role and are a major focus of research into new anti-inflammatory drugs. Such compounds include eicosanoids such as prostaglandins, prostacyclin, leukotrienes, and thromboxane A, as well as modified phospholipids such as the platelet-activating factor (PAF). Eicosanoids are synthesized from twenty-carbon polyunsaturated fatty acids by many cells, including activated leukocytes, mast cells, and platelets, and thus are widely distributed. Hormones and other inflammatory mediators (TNF-α, bradykinin) either stimulate eicosanoid production by direct PLA2 activation or indirectly by raising intracellular Ca2 + concentrations that activate the enzyme in turn. Damage to the cell membrane may also lead to increased intracellular Ca2+. Activated PLA2 immediately hydrolyzes AA, which is quickly metabolized through one of two enzyme pathways— the cyclooxygenase (COX) pathway that contributes to the formation of prostaglandin and thromboxanes, or the5-lipoxygenase (5-LOX) pathway that produces leukotrienes.

Cyclooxygenase catalyzes the oxygenation of AA in order to form the closely related cyclic endoperoxide PGG2, which is converted to PGH2. PGG2 and PGH2 are both inherently unstable and easily transformed into separate prostaglandins, prostacyclin (PGI1), and thromboxane A2 (TXA2). PGE1, PGE2, and PGI1 are active arteriolar dilators in most species ' vascular beds, which enhance the efficacy of other mediators by increasing the permeability of small veins. Other prostaglandins, which include thromboxane and PGF2α, cause smooth muscle contraction, and vasoconstriction. Prostaglandins sensitize nociceptors to pain-provoking mediators like bradykinin and histamine and can stimulate high concentrations of sensory nerve endings directly. TXA2 is a potent aggregator of platelets that participate in thrombus production.

5-LOX catalyzes the development of toxic AA hydroxy peroxides, found mainly in platelets, leukocytes, and lungs. Then, these hydroxy peroxides are converted to peptide leukotrienes. Leukotriene B4 (LTB4) and5-hydroxyeicosatetranoate (5-HETE) are strong chemoattractant that improve polymorphonuclear leucocyte movement. LTB4 also promotes the development of cytokine in neutrophils, monocytes, and eosinophils and enhances C3b receptor expression. Many leukotrienes induce the release of histamine and many autacoids from the mast cells and promote bronchiolar constriction and mucous secretion. In a few species, leukotrienes C4 and D4 are more involved in contracting the bronchial smooth muscle than histamine.

The platelet-activating factor (PAF) is also derived from PLA2 activity in the phospholipids in the cell membrane. Synthesized with mast cells, platelets, neutrophils, and eosinophils, PAF induces platelet aggregation and stimulates platelets for the development of vasoactive amines and thromboxane synthesis. PAF also increases vascular permeability and causes neutrophil aggregation and degranulation.

The function of the free radical gas Nitric Oxide in inflammation is well known. NO is an efficient cell signaling transmitter through a wide array of physiological and pathophysiological processes. Tiny amounts of NO play a part in maintaining the vascular tone resting, vasodilating, and anti-aggregating platelets. Reaction to certain cytokines (TNF-α, IL-1), and other inflammatory mediators promotes the production of relatively large amounts of NO. NO is a potent vasodilator in larger quantities, causes macrophage-induced cytotoxicity, and can contribute to joint damage in certain types of arthritis.

1.5 Symptoms of Inflammation

The inflammatory effects vary depending on whether the reaction is chronic or acute.

The acronym PRISH will describe the symptoms of acute inflammation. These include Pain: The inflamed area is likely to be painful, especially during and after the touch. They release chemicals that activate nerve endings and make the area more receptive.

Redness: This is because blood fills underlying capillaries more than average.

Immobility: Inflammatory area can cause some loss of function.

Swelling: That causes an accumulation of fluid.

Heat: More blood flows into the area affected, which makes the touch feel warm.

The five acute inflammatory signs apply only to inflammations in the skin. If inflammation happens deep inside the body, in an internal organ, for example, only some of the symptoms may be visible.

For example, few internal organs may not have neighboring sensory nerve endings, so no pain should occur, as in some types of lung inflammation.

Chronic inflammatory signs have a common form. These can include:

- Nausea
- Mouth sores
- Stomach pain
- Rash
- Joint pain

1.6 Causes of Inflammation

Inflammation is due to a number of physical reactions caused by the immune system in response to an infection or physical injury. Inflammation doesn't mean that there is an infection, but an infection may cause inflammation. Three key processes occur before and during acute inflammation: The small branches of the arteries expand as blood is transported to the affected area, resulting in increased blood flow.

Capillaries are safer for fluid and protein penetration, so they can travel between the cells and the blood.

Neutrophils discharged into the body. A neutrophil is a type of WBC filled with minuscule sacs that contain digestive enzymes and micro-organisms.

Chapter 2: Chronic Inflammation, Inflammatory Diseases and their Societal and Economic pressures

Inflammation is a critical response to possible signs of danger and damage to organs in our body.

For conditions such as rheumatoid arthritis, lupus, ulcerative colitis, Crohn's disease, and other illnesses, the immune system acts against the body's tissues. Such painful and, in some cases, slowly crippling conditions may put a toll on human quality of life and establish social and economic burdens.

Within the body, the inflammatory process plays an important function in preventing and repairing injury. It may take two basic forms, acute and chronic, commonly referred to as a cascade of inflammation, or simply an inflammation. The body's immediate response to injury or attack due to physical trauma, illness, stress, or all three combinations is acute inflammation, part of the immune response. Acute inflammation helps prevent additional damage and supports the healing and regeneration process.

Nonetheless, this can lead to chronic or long-term inflammation when inflammation becomes self-perpetuating. This is called chronic inflammation and will last beyond the actual injury; for months or even years at times. It can become a problem itself and requires medical intervention to manage or avoid further inflammation-induced damage.

Chronic inflammation may have an effect on any single body part. Also, inflammation can be a side component of many diseases. For example, in atherosclerosis or artery hardening where chronic blood vessel walls inflammation may lead to plaque build-up in the arteries, arterial or vascular blockages, and heart disease. Chronic inflammation also parts a significant role in many diseases and conditions; chronic pain, reduced sleep quality, obesity, physical disability, and decreased overall patient quality.

2.1. Societal and Economic pressures of Chronic Inflammation

Chronic inflammation may also serve as a stimulator for several carcinomas. Persistent inflammation is linked with DNA damage, which in turn can lead to cancer. For example, individuals with chronic inflammatory bowel diseases (IBD) that are Crohn's disease (CD) and ulcerative colitis (UC) have an increased risk of colon cancer. The evidence suggests that over the last three decades, there has been a dramatic increase in the number of people suffering from chronic disorders like cardiovascular diseases, diabetes, respiratory diseases, autoimmune diseases, and cancers. The increasing number of these illnesses suggests that chronic inflammation, caused by excessive and inappropriate inflammatory behavior, which in turn leads to chronic inflammatory activation in the body, may contribute to the pathology of these diseases. More evidence suggests that effective chronic inflammation therapy (i.e., reducing inflammation) can reduce the risk of cardiovascular disease.

While it is difficult to measure the actual economic impact of chronic inflammation since it spreads to almost all areas of chronic disease, certain common chronic inflammation-mediated diseases can be investigated. For example, Direct healthcare costs incurred in Europe by IBD-affected patients were estimated at € 4.6–5.6 billion per year.

Health inequalities in chronic inflammatory diseases are widespread; Black Americans, for example, are 3 to 4 times more likely to have chronic kidney disease-related morbidity and mortality than white Americans.

The expense of chronic obstructive pulmonary disease (COPD) in the US was estimated at about $50 billion in 2010, including $30 billion in direct health care expenditures and $20 billion in indirect spending. The combined direct and indirect costs of UK

Economic Burden NHS due to COPD were calculated at £ 982 million. In Europe, the annual cost of treating COPD is estimated at € 38.6 billion.

Chronic diseases may worsen depression symptoms and even depressive disorders, leading to chronic diseases.

2.2. Rheumatoid Arthritis

Rheumatoid arthritis is a chronic inflammatory condition (possibly affecting the entire body) that usually affects the small joints in the hands and feet. RA is an inflammatory disease in which a person's immune system attacks joint tissues and probably other body parts/organs for unexplained reasons. Symptoms can spread as the disease progresses to the wrists, knees, ankles, elbows, hips, and shoulders. Consequently, RA causes the joints to suffer from discomfort, inflammation and ultimately damage and malformation. RA may cause people to feel ill, exhausted, and feverish; it also symmetrically affects joints where the pain in the joint is felt on both sides of the body.17- RA is markedly different from osteoarthritis (OA), a degenerative joint disease that only limits joint function. However, pediatric arthritis and rheumatological disorders have affected approximately 294,000 children under the age of 18 in the US. The most common age of onset among women is between 30 and 60 years, whereas it occurs later in men's lives. Per-patient costs for uninsured Rheumatoid Arthritis patients were estimated at $5,758, which is aggregated to an annual total expense of $560 million when weighted by uninsured prevalence. In the United Kingdom, the National Audit Office (NAO) found that in 2009, RA cost about £560 million per year to the National Health Service (NHS), with the majority of this spending in the acute sector, and that the total expense was calculated at around £560 million per year.

Studies show that an increase in early treatment for RA patients would bring significant productivity benefits, with economic gains of £ 31 m due to decreased sick leave and job losses. According to the NAO of the United Kingdom, 10 percent of RA patients are treated within three months of the onset of symptoms; economic analysis suggests that increasing this to 20 percent can cause cost increases, but faster treatment may become cost-neutral after nearly nine years.

2.3. Psoriatic Arthritis

Psoriatic arthritis is an inflammatory arthritis type that can sometimes be serious, a chronic, autoimmune disease. Nearly 30 per cent of chronic skin psoriasis patients will also develop psoriatic arthritis. Patients with PSA inflammation will also experience painful swelling in hand and wrist joints. In addition, PSA may also develop this type of psoriatic arthritis. Many patients also experience physical disabilities due to their PSA, reduced emotional well-being and general tiredness. This in turn leads to direct medical costs from the use of health care services. The resulting functional limitations lead to indirect costs such as disability and lost productivity, and are significant drivers of total care costs. In the US, the direct annual health care costs for PSA are estimated to be as high as $1.9 billion, based on an average cost per patient of $3,638.36. A European analysis found a total direct cost of $4,008 in Hungary.

2.4. Inflammatory Bowel Disease (IBD), ulcerative colitis (UC) and Crohn's disease (CD)

Inflammatory intestinal disease (IBD) identifies disorders of chronic or persistent immune response and gastrointestinal (GI) tract inflammation. Ulcerative colitis (UC) and Crohn's disease (CD) are the two most common inflammatory bowel diseases.

UC mainly affects the large intestine, while any part of the GI tract may be affected by CD. Symptoms of UC often include blood and mucus-containing diarrhea, severe cramp-like abdominal pain, anemia, loss of appetite, weight loss, fatigue, strong bowel movement desire, and tenesmus (incomplete evacuation sensation). Individuals with moderate to severe UC reported negative effects on education, jobs, social/personal life, relationships, and depression. Surveys have shown anxiety and stress that people with UC complain about their disease. More than seventy percent of people with UC have reported symptoms affecting their ability to enjoy leisure activities, and nearly two-thirds report their symptoms of UC influencing their work performance. About 1.6 million Americans have IBD, an increase of around 200,000 since this statistic was last recorded by the Crohn's and Colitis Foundation of America in 2011.

Up to 70,000, new cases of IBD are diagnosed annually in the United States. In the United States, there could be as many as 80,000 children with IBD.44 In 2012, there were nearly 233,000 Canadians living with IBD (129,000 persons with CD and 104,000 persons with (UC). An approximate 2,5–3 million people in Europe suffer from IBD. In Asia, we are seeing growing incidence of IBD. Thirty years ago, with IBD, Hong Kong was home to less than 1 in 1 million people. Today about 3 out of 100,000 people in Hong Kong are diagnosed with new IBDs.

2.5. Chronic obstructive pulmonary disease (COPD)

Chronic pulmonary obstructive disease (COPD) develops as an effective, chronic

Half of COPD patients face movement restrictions due to health problems compared to 17 percent of patients without COPD. Many people with COPD (38%) report having difficulty walking or climbing stairs, compared to those without the condition (11%). Many people with COPD (22 percent) claim they need to use special equipment for health problems compared with 7 percent without COPD among adults. COPD is the third-most-common cause of death in the United States. It is estimated 3 million people in the United Kingdom suffer from COPD. And the disease kills about 30,000 people a year, more than breast, bowel, or penile cancer. France has 3.5 million COPD sufferers (6 percent adult incidence) and 16,000 deaths every year.

2.6. Treatment of Chronic Inflammation

Although acute inflammation is part of the animal body's natural system of protection against injury and disease, chronic inflammation in itself is considered a disease. Because chronic inflammation affects specific areas of the body and can be associated with a defined disease process, treatment approaches vary considerably.49 Physicians have relied on steroids for decades to suppress immune response. Steroids, though an effective choice, come with common side effects such as weight gain and potentially harmful side effects such as heart enlargement and liver cancer. Today, as science has progressed, new classes of therapies have been developed which transform inflammatory disease management by targeting other main proteins and body pathways. Today, patients with chronic inflammation and inflammatory disease have new treatment choices with more targeted agents that go beyond wide-ranging immunosuppressive therapies.

Scientists' ability to better understand the underlying biology of the disease and identify groups of patients can lead to new and innovative medicines through precision medicine, which will best respond to certain treatments.

Chapter 3: Arthritis is an Inflammatory Disease

Inflammatory arthritis is a phrase used to describe a group of conditions that affect the immune system. This means that your body's defense system starts attacking your own tissues rather than germs, viruses, and other foreign substances that can cause pain, stiffness, and joint damage. These are also known for being autoimmune diseases. Inflammatory arthritis has three most common forms: rheumatoid arthritis, ankylosing spondylitis, psoriatic arthritis. These illnesses are also called systemic diseases since they can affect the whole body. They can happen at any age.

Such diseases are still not healed, but the outlook for those afflicted with inflammatory arthritis is much better than it was 20–30 years ago. Effective treatment begins much earlier, and new drugs are available, which means less joint damage, less need for surgery, and fewer complications.

Inflammatory arthritis is not the same as osteoarthritis that happens when the cartilage inside the joint is rubbed away.

The inflammatory arthritis route is a guide to what information is available and could be of help to you at any major point of your journey, from first detected symptoms to specialist care if the disease progresses. The route guides you through each process to relevant organizations and sources of information.

Steps to Arthritic Pathway

<u>Step 1–Recognizing symptoms prior to seeking medical help</u>

You can experience joint and/or back pain at Step 1, but your GP has not yet looked at the symptoms. You might have seen a few of the following two posters warning individuals of one of the three most severe types of inflammatory arthritis: rheumatoid arthritis, ankylosing spondylitis, and psoriatic arthritis.

The Squeeze Test is the most common measure for rheumatoid arthritis and psoriatic arthritis that includes pushing the patient's hand or foot across the knuckle joints, as shown. If this examination is unduly painful, then there may be signs of those conditions.

Test A gives an MCP (metacarpophalangeal) test.

Test B shows an MTP (Metatarsophalangeal) test.

If you have signs that may be associated with inflammatory arthritis, don't delay and seek help from your GP as soon as possible.

Phase 2–First time visiting the doctor:

At Step 2, you'll see your doctor first. The following links will help with your first GP visit, handle your symptoms, and get general health advice. There is also some information that you might find helpful while waiting for your first specialist appointment, which should be within 4–6 weeks.

Inflammatory arthritis can, at times, be difficult to diagnose, and usually, only a rheumatologist specialist or a GP with a specific interest in musculoskeletal disorder (GPWSI) may make a firm diagnosis. Since the various causes of inflammatory arthritis are treated by specialist teams led by a rheumatologist doctor and are usually hospital-based, but not always, this is a specialized treatment area. This means that they may not have the level of experience, skill, and knowledge needed to make a clinical diagnosis unless your GP has been qualified to be a specialist in addition.

There's no one test that you can take to tell if you're getting rheumatoid arthritis, ankylosing spondylitis, or psoriatic arthritis, so it's essential that if your GP feels you're having either of those disorders, they'll refer you to a rheumatologist specialist for assessment as soon as possible.

The British Pain Society has a number of articles on pain management with in-depth advice.

The NHS Live Well pages offer general health recommendations on a variety of topics, including healthy eating, smoking cessation, and exercise.

The Patients Association has a number of manuals, including one entitled *Preparing the GP for an appointment."

Your first specialist appointment should be within four to six weeks, but it may be quicker if the waiting times in your area allow.

Phase 3–First seeing the doctor after referral:

You should see the doctor at Phase 3 (most definitely a physician for rheumatology) first. You may get a solid diagnosis during your first visit, but in the very early stages, it is sometimes difficult to diagnose inflammatory arthritis. If you have rheumatoid arthritis, ankylosing spondylitis, or psoriatic arthritis, no single test will tell you, so for diagnosis, and you may need more tests and visits.

The links below will help you with this phase in your path and will guide you to other organizations that can provide more information. It includes information about: your first medical meeting and how to make potential treatment plans for the healthcare professionals who may be interested in your treatment.

Using NICE recommendations (RA) is meant to help you understand the care and treatment facilities that should be provided in the NHS for those with rheumatoid arthritis.

We suggest you think and take note of everything you want to know before your first visit to see the expert. This will help ensure the answer to all your questions during the consultation process. It may also be helpful to have a friend or family member with you, as they may remember stuff you did not take in afterward.

Step 4–Testing, procedures and additional information

You will get your first diagnosis at Phase 4, and search for appropriate care with your specialist team. At this stage, you might need to have a number of tests to help your specialist team decide the best treatment for you. These tests could include x-ray ultrasound scans for blood test Disease activity scores. These tests may seem a bit confusing to start with, particularly when you've just been diagnosed, but your rheumatology nurse practitioner will help explain them to you on your first visit. During your first or second doctor visit, you will usually meet the rheumatology nurse practitioner. The qualified nurse will help answer a few of your possible questions.

Step 5–Continuing care in primary and specialist care:

Treatment will continue at Phase 5. You will usually see your team of specialists very often to start with, but your visits will become less regular once your team is confident that your condition is well handled.

With regular blood tests, you will need to go to your GP surgery or the hospital. These will check how you manage the disorder and how you respond to the therapy. Then, the GP will speak to the specialist team about some of the diagnosis.

You and your family will be revisiting the disease and its effects on your life at least once a year when your condition is in balance.

If you have a problem or an increase in your symptoms, it's important that you know how to get in touch. You should get access to a nurse-led helpline call.

As well as the organizations mentioned below that include person-specific information in Step 5, you may also be interested in the following general information: The Patients Association is an independent, national charity that addresses the issues and needs of patients.

The Citizens Advice Bureau offers information on health rights, which includes what assistance is available via the NHS, patient rights, health cost aid, how to make a complaint, and health care for people abroad.

Direct Government defines the assistance that may be provided across a number of topics such as education, transportation, and finance.

Most specialty teams have a line of instruction often run by the specialist nurse-making sure you know the number. Your GP is also a reliable source of aid and support.

Phase 6-Managing the long-term illness or coping with complications:

Phase 6 is an advanced disorder, affecting only a few individuals. Advanced illness may include organs such as your heart and lungs that can cause severe complications and/or other long-term conditions such as diabetes or heart disease. Other complications can rarely occur like vasculitis.

However, for those dealing with inflammatory arthritis, the situation today is significantly better than it was 20–30 years ago. Despite significant new therapies now available, and effective treatment started much earlier than it used to be, with less discomfort, less need for surgery, and fewer complications, the future is much brighter. The better you know, and how to handle your condition.

The links below give information about possible complications. You can also identify specific organizations that can assist you, including those that offer assistance to caregivers.

Chapter 4: Gastritis an Inflammatory disease – Causes, signs and symptoms, treatment and cure

Gastritis is an inflammation of a stomach lining. There are two types of acute gastritis, and a chronic one. Most people with gastritis may have no symptoms; however, both acute and chronic gastritis may have symptoms and signs of abdominal pain, diarrhea, vomiting, and sometimes belching, bloating, loss of appetite, and indigestion.

What causes an upset stomach?

A bacterium known as Helicobacter pylori and non-steroidal anti-inflammatory drugs are the major cause of gastritis, and there are many other causes of the condition too, such as infectious agents, autoimmune disorders, illnesses such as Crohn's disease, sarcoidosis, and sporadic granulomatosis gastritis. How do you know if you feel upset about your stomach?

Gastritis may be diagnosed either by examining the symptoms and history (e.g., NSAID and/or alcohol) or by testing breath, blood, urine, immunology, and biopsy for H. Pylori and other measures such as endoscopy or radiological studies show improvements in the mucosa.

4.1. Some facts about gastritis

What is Treatment for Gastritis?
Treatment with gastritis varies by source. Other less common causes may receive similar treatment, but do not address the underlying cause.

Is there a diet on gastritis?
Symptoms of gastritis can be worsened by chemical irritants, which should reduce or avoid the gastritis symptoms together. Stop smoking cigarettes, for example, reduce excessive alcohol consumption, avoid caffeinated, decaffeinated, and carbonated drinks; and fruit juices containing citric acid, such as grapefruit, peach, pineapple, etc., and avoid high-fat foods.

There is no diet for gastritis, however, and the growth of H. A diet rich in fiber and foods containing flavonoids such as certain teas, onions, garlic, berries, celery, kale, broccoli, parsley, thyme, soy products, and legumes such as lentils, kidney, green, wheat, pinto, and marine beans can prevent pylori.

Which home remedies help to ease the symptoms of gastritis?

Home remedies may help to reduce gastritis symptoms, but normally the underlying cause of the condition is not handled.

Individuals suffering from acute gastritis usually recover without complications. However, if serious complications arise, there could be a variety of results from good (early treatment) to poor for chronic gastritis. Acute gastritis complications may occur very rarely.

Chronic gastritis complications include peptic ulcer, bleeding ulcers, anemia, stomach cancers, MALT lymphoma, renal issues, tightness, intestinal inflammation, or even death.

Gastritis may also be prevented if the underlying causes of gastritis (e.g., alcohol use or use of NSAIDs) are treated or not used. Is one possible cure for gastritis?

Gastritis can be treated if it treats the cause that underlies it.

Why do you fight gastritis?

Since gastritis is an infection and can be avoided by washing your hands thoroughly and often, for example, using good hand washing techniques, avoid circumstances where you are exposed to chemical substances, radiation, or toxins in order to avoid gastritis risk.

What foods light up gastritis symptoms?

Health care professionals at Maryland University and others say eating smaller, more frequent meals and avoiding salty, acidic, fried, or fatty foods will help reduce symptoms. In fact, a reduction of stress is also advised. Dietary improvements such as ginger tea and/or honey chamomile tea allegedly relieve gastritis symptoms while H can be prevented by onions, garlic, cranberries, apples, and celery. Pylori Production.

Foods that might hamper H. Pylori growth and relief of gastritis symptoms include teas (particularly green and white) Yogurt, Peppermint, Wheat bran, Carrot juice, Coconut, water Green leafy vegetables, Onions, Garlic, Apples, Fresh fruits and berries Celery Cranberry juice, Kale, Broccoli, Scallions Parsley, Thyme, Soybeans, cSoy foods Legumes (beans, peas, and lentils). Although these home remedies can help reduce or soothe symptoms,

4.2. Causes of gastritis

Stomach mucosal infection by a bacterial species called Helicobacter pylori is a major cause of both acute as well as chronic gastritis. This bacterium usually initially acutely infects the stomach antrum (stomach mucosa without acid-producing cells) and may grow over time to infect most or all of the stomach mucosa (chronic gastritis) and remain there for years. This infection triggers an initial strong inflammatory response, and with changes in the intestinal cells, long-term chronic inflammation can eventually develop. Another main cause of acute and chronic gastritis is the use (and overuse) of non-steroidal anti-inflammatory drugs (NSAIDs).

Nevertheless, there are many other causes of gastritis; the following is a list of common causes of both acute and chronic gastritis; with repeated or persistent presence of most of these causes, chronic gastritis may occur: bacterial, viral and parasite infections.

4.3. Symptoms of gastritis

Most patients suffering from gastritis are without symptoms. The condition is only reported when other possible diseases are checked for the stomach mucosal samples. Nevertheless, as signs of gastritis develop, the most common symptoms are abdominal pain (intermittent or constant burning, squeezing or gnawing pain), nausea and vomiting, diarrhea, loss of appetite, bloating, burping, and belching.

Symptoms of gastritis come and go through time, particularly with chronic gastritis. Indigestion (dyspepsia) is also another concept that involves this cluster of symptoms. Symptoms of extreme gastritis may include prolonged diarrhea, bloody stools, and anemia.

4.4. Natural remedies for gastritis

Not all therapies would work for everyone, so a person might have to try out several of these before they find out what works best for their situation.

1. Follow an anti-inflammatory diet: Gastritis is also considered as inflammation of the stomach lining and eating a diet that can provide relief over time to help reduce inflammation. Nevertheless, research has not shown conclusively that gastritis is caused or avoided by eating a certain diet.

By keeping a dietary diary, people may recognize which foods cause their symptoms. We can then start to reduce their intake or avoid other foods altogether.

Foods commonly associated with inflammation are: processed foods gluten acidic foods Milky foods Spicy alcohol foods

2. Consume a garlic extract supplement: Some research suggests that garlic extract can help lower the symptoms of gastritis. Crushing and consuming raw garlic will also work well.

If a person does not like the raw taste of garlic, they might try to chop the garlic and eat it with a spoonful of peanut butter or wrapped in on a dry date. The sweet taste of the peanut butter, or date, should help mask the garlic flavor.

3. Probiotics: Probiotics can help improve digestion and facilitate regular bowel movements. Probiotic additives introduce good bacteria into a person's digestive tract that can help stop H spread.

Eating foods that contain probiotics can also improve the symptoms of gastritis. Such foods include kimchi kombucha sauerkraut kefir yogurt.

4. Drink some green, honey tea manuka. One study showed that consuming green or black tea can reduce the prevalence of H substantially, at least once a week. Gastrointestinal Pylori. Manuka honey may also be useful in that it contains antibacterial properties that help fight infection.

Many people believe warm drinking water soothes the stomach and improves digestion.

Manuka honey can be purchased online and in health-care shops.

5. Use of essential oils: Essential oils such as lemongrass and lemon verbena have been found to help improve resistance to H. Pylori in laboratory work.

Few other oils that can have a positive effect on the digestive system are peppermint, ginger, and clove.

Essential oils should not be engulfed and should always be diluted with a carrier oil when applied to the skin.

Users might want to use the oils in a diffuser or talk to a doctor about using them safely to help relieve gastritis.

It's important to remember that the AMERICAN Food and Drug Administration (FDA) does not authorize natural oils or herbal medicine.

6. Eat lighter meals: eating large, heavy carbohydrate meals can put a strain on the digestive system of a person and make gastritis worse. Eating small meals regularly during the day can help ease the digestive process and reduce the symptoms of gastritis.

7. Avoid smoking and extra use of painkillers: smoking can harm a person's stomach lining, and it also increases the chances of developing cancer in the stomach.

Taking too many pain medications over - the counter, including aspirin or ibuprofen, can also weaken the stomach lining and make gastritis even worse.

8. Reduce stress: Stress can produce gastritis flare-ups, so rising stress levels is an effective way to help manage the disease.

Strategies for stress management include Relaxation breathing exercises, sleep therapy, and yoga.

Prevention: While the cause of gastritis differs between people, certain precautions may be taken to avoid unpleasant symptoms.

Steps to reduce gastritis include: avoiding known triggering foods to stop smoking influence and reducing the stress that prevents alcohol from maintaining a healthy weight that prevents overuse-the-counter pain medications Home remedies can help many people manage gastritis. However, when symptoms do not go away, it is necessary to talk to a doctor. When to see a doctor, Patients with gastritis should see a doctor if they experience: a gastritis flare-up that lasts longer than a week, vomiting blood in the stool. A doctor may ask questions, conduct an evaluation, and may decide to perform other tests.

Common gastritis prescribed medicines include histamine blockers 2 (H2), which help to reduce the production of acid. Proton pump inhibitors (PPIs) are available in both prescription and over - the counter forms, which also work to decreases acid production and are available on the counter as well as on prescription antibiotics used to treat H. Pylori Infection.

Chapter 5: Anti-inflammatory Dietary Tips for Gastritis

Gastritis is a digestive disease that causes the stomach lining to become inflamed. Symptoms include heartburn, indigestion, diarrhea, and frequent burping. A few people will benefit from dietary changes. Gastritis has various forms and causes. Infection with Helicobacter pylori bacteria (H. pylori) is one common cause. Other causes include the use of non-steroidal anti-inflammatory drugs (NSAIDs), high intake of alcohol, and certain inflammatory disorders, such as Crohn's disease.

Some foods can add to the risk of H. Pylori infection, and certain dietary habits can cause stomach lining erosion or otherwise aggravate gastritis symptoms. A person suffering from gastritis can find eating hard, leading to loss of appetite and unwanted weight loss.

Untreated gastritis can lead to ulceration, chronic pain, and bleeding. In some cases, it can turn life-threatening. Chronic stomach inflammation also increases stomach cancer development.

5.1. Anti-inflammatory Foods to eat

No particular diet can cure gastritis, but eating certain foods can help improve or prevent the symptoms from getting worse.

Dietary changes, for example, can help protect the stomach lining and reduce inflammation.

Green tea and fresh fruits and vegetables can help to prevent gastritis in the body. They are good sources of antioxidants and can help to prevent cell damage and disease by raising the levels of reactive compounds called free radicals in the body. Aliments that may help inhibit development of H. Pylori and reduced gastritis and ulcer growth include cauliflower, swede, cabbage, radish, and other Brassica vegetable berries, such as turmeric blueberries, blackberries, raspberries, and strawberries; a mild spice that may have anti-inflammatory properties Antioxidants may also help prevent a wide range of other conditions. There you can learn more about antioxidants and the foods they include. Foods that help alleviate Gastritis symptoms include stomach lining inflammation. For this reason, an anti-inflammatory diet may be beneficial to some people.

There's no ideal anti-inflammatory diet. Eat plenty of antioxidant-rich fresh fruit, vegetables, and other plant foods to combat inflammation. It is more important to avoid processed foods and those containing unhealthy fats and to add salt or sugar.

Foods to help treat gastritis: Broccoli and yogurt are two foods that can help with gastritis care.

Broccoli contains a chemical sulforaphane which has antibacterial properties. It also includes antioxidants that can aid in the prevention of cancer. Consequently, eating broccoli sprouts can help relieve or prevent gastritis and reduce the risk of stomach cancer. An older study published in 2009 by scientists has identified participants with H. Pylori infections that ate 70 grams of broccoli sprouts per day — more than half a cup — had lower infection and inflammation levels for eight weeks than those that didn't eat broccoli.

In 2006, another team investigated whether eating around 2 cups of probiotic yogurt a day before using an antibiotic combination could improve the ability of the medication to combat drug-resistant H. Pylori. Yeah.

After four weeks, the researchers found that people who drank yogurt and antibiotics tended to kill the infection more effectively than those who just took antibiotics. The findings in the yogurt may have been obtained from the active cultures of beneficial bacteria that help improve the body's ability to fight infection.

5.2. Dietary Tips

The following dietary changes will help prevent or regulate gastritis: Eat little but often: eating five to six smaller meals throughout the day— instead of three big meals — can help reduce the accumulation of stomach acids.

Managing weight: Overweight and obesity increase the risk of developing gastritis. A doctor can help create a weight loss plan to reduce the risk of gastritis and other associated health issues.

Use antacids: A doctor may also advise on pain relief drugs.

Ask a Physician about supplements: some dietary supplements, including omega-3 fatty acids and probiotics, can reduce the effects of gastritis.

Omega-3 antioxidants and probiotic supplements can be ordered online. Still, talk to a doctor before taking these or other supplements, as they may interfere with other health issues.

Additionally, some additives, including iron, can increase the risk of gastritis. Foods that make symptoms worse include: spicy fried foods that are acidic in alcohol can sometimes cause an allergen to inflammation. In this type of case, a doctor might recommend a diet for elimination, which includes removing all food groups from the diet to see if it causes the symptoms.

One team of doctors, for example, reported that one person has a form of gastritis caused by dairy and egg. The team also had been looking at wheat, nuts, soy, fish, and rice.

Those considering an elimination diet should first speak to a physician, as it may cause nutritional deficiencies.

Foods that increase the risk of gastritis: if a person consumes: red meat processed meat products that are alcohol-pickled, fried, salted, or smoked fatty foods, Studies have shown that, for example, salty and fatty foods can affect the stomach lining. High-salt diets can change the cells within the stomach, making them more susceptible to H. Pylori.

High levels of alcohol can also cause stomach inflammation and worsen the symptoms. It can also induce an erode in the stomach lining.

Any health tips: Stop smoking to help with gastritis prevention or treatment: smoking increases the risk of inflammation, teeth, esophageal, and stomach cancer.

Reducing stress: High levels of stress can cause stomach acid to develop, which can aggravate symptoms and inflammation.

Checking any medication: Frequent use of NSAIDs may increase the risk of damage to the stomach lining, which may cause or worsen symptoms of gastritis. The aspirin, ibuprofen, and naproxen are all forms of NSAID.

5.3. Diet for stomach ulcers and gastritis

A diet of ulcer and gastritis is a meal plan that restricts foods that irritate your stomach. Most products have the ability to worsen symptoms such as stomach pain, bloating, heartburn, or indigestion.

<u>Foods: will I limit or avoid</u>? You might need to avoid acidic, spicy, or high-fat foods. Not every food has the same effect on everybody. You'll need to learn which foods exacerbate the symptoms and limit other foods. Some foods that could worsen the symptoms of ulcer or gastritis are as follows: beverages, whole milk, chocolate milk, Hot cocoa, and cola. Some drinks with caffeine Regular and decaffeinated coffee Peppermint and spearmint tea Green and black tea, with or without caffeine Orange and grapefruit juices. Eat whole grains, nuts, vegetables, and dairy products that are free of fat or low in fat, includes bread of whole wheat, cereals, noodles, and brown rice—select lean meats, poultry, fish, beans, nuts, and vegetables. A healthy meal plan includes low unhealthy fat levels, salt, and added sugar.

Healthy fats come from canola and olive oil. Consult a healthy meal plan with your dietitian for more.

What could further guidance help?

Do not feed only prior to bedtime. Arrange for feeding at least 2 hours prior to bedtime.

Eat small and daily meals. Small, regular meals can be more accommodating to your stomach than big meals.

Procedure AGREEMENT: You have the right to help with the planning of the procedure. To decide what care you want to get, speak with your doctor about treatment options. Yours is also the right to deny medication. The above knowledge is a pure educational aid. Talk to your GP, nurse, or pharmacist before taking any medical treatment to see if it's safe and effective for you.

Chapter 6: Obesity and Inflammation are interrelated

Obesity is a health issue that has reached widespread proportions with growing global prevalence. The global obesity epidemic increases the risk of chronic metabolic disorders. It is, therefore, an economic problem that increased the costs of the related comorbidities. Moreover, obesity has been shown to be associated with chronic systemic inflammation in recent years, and this status is caused by innate activation of the immune system in adipose tissue, which promotes increased production and release of pro-inflammatory cytokines that lead to the systemic acute-phase response characterized by elevation of acute cytokines. Therefore, a growing body of evidence confirms the important role played by the inflammatory response in obesity condition and the related pathogenesis of chronic diseases.

6.1. Obesity and Chronic Inflammation

Inflammation is a physiological response needed to restore homeostasis, which is altered by various stimuli; however, inflammation or excessive response that is permanently established may have deleterious effects. In overweight and obesity, low-grade chronic inflammation exists; recent studies have identified some of the intracellular inflammation pathways associated with these conditions; experiments in mice and humans show that the ingestion of nutrients acutely activates inflammatory responses; thus, it is believed that the starting signal of inflammation is overfeeding and that the pathway originates In ob. These kinases control downstream transcriptional programs by inducing regulation of the expression of the inflammatory mediator gene through transcription factors protein-1 activator, nuclear factor πB, and interferon regulator. The increase in cytokines exacerbates the activation of receptors by creating a positive inflammatory feedback loop and signaling the inhibitory metabolic pathways.

Inflammasomal and Toll-like receptors (TLRs) likewise activate the innate immune system. Strong evidence now suggests that inflammatory signaling plays a prominent role in developing a chronic inflammatory disorder that impairs insulin responsiveness.

6.2. The Inflammasome

The inflammasome is a sensor of the innate macromolecular immune cells which activate the inflammatory response.

Recognition of various noxious signals by the inflammasome results in the activation of caspase-1, which then induces the secretion of potent proinflammatory cytokines, in particular interleukin-1β (IL-1β). In this way, inflammasome-mediated processes are important for the regulation of metabolic processes.

The inflammasome is a heptamer assembled from monomers containing Nod-like receptors (NLRs), the ASC adapter protein (an apoptosis-associated speck-like protein containing a caspase-recruitment domain), and the caspase-1 enzyme. NLRs are distinguished by a structure composed of a central realm that mediates nucleotide-binding and oligomerization and a variable N terminal area essential for protein-protein interactions. The NLR activates caspase-1, which, when assembled as an inflammasome, converts pro-IL-1β into active IL-1β.

The NLR family is made up of 22 members for humans, divided into four subfamilies, NLRA, NLRB, NLRC, and NLRP, based on their N-terminal domain configuration. We interact with the inflammasome-related proteins ASC and caspase-1. Metabolic tension, insulin resistance, and type 2 diabetes have been associated with an NLRP member named NLRP3. Inflammatory activation of NLRP3 in obesity induces macrophage-mediated activation of T cells in adipose tissue and impairs insulin sensitivity establishing a persistent pro-inflammatory condition that impairs the sensitivity of insulins. Among other substances, hyperglycemia, reactive oxygen species, palmitate, lipopolysaccharides, and uric acid can cause inflammasome activation.

Recent studies have shown that a glucose-upregulated protein, the protein that interacts with thioredoxin (TXNIP), interacts with NLRP3, resulting in IL-1β secretion and pancreatic β-cell function impairment.

6.3. The Inflammatory Cytokines and Obesity

The cause of the inflammation during obesity and the underlying molecular mechanisms causing its prevalence are not fully understood, but pro-inflammatory cytokines play a central role. In obesity, inflammatory cytokines show higher circulating concentrations than in lean beings, and they are believed to play a role in insulin resistance induction. The adipose tissue is the primary source of pro-inflammatory cytokines in obesity; it is released primarily through macrophage infiltration, while adipocytes play a role. Thus, the blood levels of these cytokines are reduced after weight loss. The main cytokines responsible for chronic inflammation are the tumor necrosis factor-αγ, interleukin-6, and the inflammasome-activated IL-1β.

TNF-α is a pleiotropic molecule that parts a central role in inflammation, immune system production, apoptosis, and lipid metabolism, having numerous effects in adipose tissue, including lipid metabolism and insulin signaling — circulating TNF-α increases in obesity and declines in weight loss. TNF-α stimulates IL-6 release, another strong pro-inflammatory cytokine, and reduces anti-inflammatory cytokines such as adiponectin. TNF-α induces adipocyte apoptosis and encourages insulin resistance by inhibiting a signaling pathway for the insulin receptor substratum.

It is a cytokine that plays significant roles in the development of acute phase reactions, inflammation, hematopoiesis, metabolism of the bone, and cancer. It controls energy homeostasis and inflammation; it may inhibit the production of lipoprotein lipase, and influences hypothalamic appetite and energy intake is important for the transition from acute to chronic inflammatory disease. For conditions such as obesity, insulin resistance, inflammatory intestinal disease, inflammatory arthritis, and sepsis, this leads to chronic inflammation when deregulated.

IL-1β is a pyrogenic cytokine. It is primarily developed by blood monocytes as a response to infection, injury, or immunological threat; this causes fever, hypotension, and the production of additional pro-inflammatory cytokines such as IL-6. IL-1β is formed from its pro-IL-1β inactive counterpart by an inflammasome. But IL-1β has now emerged as a leading instigator of the pro-inflammatory response to obesity. Significant progress has been made in the last decade in understanding the role of cytokines and the inflammasome in obesity, chronic inflammation, and type 2 diabetes. Also, further work is needed to better understand the underlying mechanisms, since they are possible points of intervention in the quest for new therapeutic modalities for these global health problems.

6.4. Markers of Inflammation in Obesity

Many chronic diseases include an inflammatory response marked by a rise in cytokines and serum concentrations of acute-phase reactants such as fibrinogen, C-reactive protein (CRP), complement, serum amyloid A, haptoglobin, sialic acid and low concentrations of albumin. Acute-phase reactants are made in the liver, and cytokines, includingIL-6 and TNF-alpha, regulate its production. Considered the classic sensitive acute-phase reactant, the CRP is a very sensitive systemic inflammation marker, and its serum concentration is rapidly increasing as a response to a variety of stimuli. Under normal conditions, this protein is found in low concentrations.

Visceral adipose tissue can generate inflammatory mediators that cause acute-phase reactants to be generated in hepatocytes and endothelial cells. Perhaps because adipocytes have been shown to express and secrete TNF-alpha, adipose body mass may be an important mediator in understanding the relationship between obesity and inflammation. Several studies have shown that abdominal adiposity is correlated with CRP level elevation, independent of the body mass index (BMI), which is a general adiposity scale. In those individuals with abdominal adiposity, the proportion of people with elevated hs-CRP was significantly higher than control subjects, although they had a comparable BMI. This is a pro-inflammatory cytokine synthesized with adipose, endothelial, macrophage, and lymphocyte tissue. In the liver, the CRP is mainly synthesized in response to IL-6 stimuli. Obese people are at increased risk for multiple chronic diseases, of which several are often distinguished by high concentrations of CRP. Because adipose tissue is the main component of pro-inflammatory cytokines such as IL-6and TNF-alpha, both cytokines increase lipogenesis in the hepatic and cause a systemic acute-phase response.

In recent years, obesity has been shown to be associated with low-grade inflammatory processes characterized by elevated circulating levels of pro-inflammatory cytokines in healthy obese subjects such as IL-6, TNF-alpha, and acute-phase proteins (CRP and haptoglobin). This pattern is also seen in obese children who have higher levels of CRP than children with average weights. Some studies have indicated that dietary weight loss is associated with decreased circulating levels of IL-6, TNF-alpha, CRP, and other inflammation markers regardless of age, sex, and BMI. Likewise, the weight reduction observed after gastric bypass in subjects indicates a decrease in rates of CRP andIL-6.

6.5. Metabolic Syndrome

The metabolic syndrome has three or more of the following characteristics: obesity, hyperglycemia, hypertension, low HDL cholesterol levels, and/or hypertriglyceridemia. While pathogenic mechanisms are poorly understood, a central role has been assigned to the pro-inflammatory cytokine's TNF-alpha and IL-6, as both are synthesized by adipose tissue. Inflammatory activity factors such as CRP, IL-6, serum amyloid

A and soluble adhesion molecules have been associated with this condition.

Risk factors: Low-grade chronic inflammation is consistent with metabolic syndrome, and some features of insulin resistance. Several studies have shown a substantial association of CRP levels with symptoms of metabolic syndrome, including adiposity, hyperinsulinemia, resistance to insulin, hypertriglyceridemia, and low cholesterol HDL. In just a few studies, the relationship between CRP and the development of metabolic syndrome has been established. In addition, elevated levels of hs-CRP have been shown to be associated with having metabolic syndrome with increased risk of adverse cardiovascular events in individuals. Inflammation was proposed as a common part of various metabolic disturbances of insulin, glucose, and lipids affecting the underlying development of the metabolic syndrome.

It has also shown that CRP has independent prognostic information on the extent of metabolic syndrome. It has been suggested that CRP is an additional component of metabolic syndrome. In one research, it was explained that elevated CRP levels (almost 3 mg / L) might increase the risk of metabolic syndrome caused by factors of obesity and resistance to insulin.

Healing counseling: Observational studies have shown that dietary patterns close to the Mediterranean diet, rich in fruits and vegetables, and high in monounsaturated fiber and fats, have resulted in reduced prevalence of metabolic syndromes. Furthermore, interventional studies have also shown a decrease in inflammatory factors following Mediterranean diets and/or national dietary guidelines in subjects with metabolic syndrome.

Work to assess inflammation pathways in individuals with metabolic syndrome is scarce; however, some have reported anti-inflammatory effects from statin therapy. Since subjects with metabolic syndrome show increased inflammation, statins may be a therapeutic alternative following improvement in the lifestyle of therapy.

6.6. Chronic Inflammation and Metabolic Syndrome

The rising incidence of obesity and metabolic syndrome is worrying. The activation of inflammatory pathways, typically used as a defense for the host, causes the severity of this illness. Inflammation activation is most likely more than one cause. Evidently, metabolic overload evokes stress responses, such as oxidative, inflammatory, organelle, and cell hypertrophy, leading to vicious cycles. For physical reasons, adipocyte hypertrophy causes cell separation and will cause an inflammatory reaction. The inability to grow adipose tissue to absorb incoming fat leads to deposition in other organs with effects on insulin resistance, especially in the liver. The oxidative stress that accompanies eating may contribute to the inflammation that is associated with obesity, particularly when fat and/or other macronutrients are overly ingested without the concomitant ingestion of antioxidant-rich foods/beverages. Furthermore, work on the interaction of microbiota with food and obesity brought with its new hypothesis for the relationship between obesity / fat diet and inflammation. Some causes, such as shifts in the psychological and/or circadian rhythms, may also result in oxidative/inflammatory status beyond these. The challenge of treating obesity / metabolic syndrome is due to its multifactorial existence, where environmental, genetic, and psychosocial causes interact through complex networks.

Metabolic syndrome prevalence increases and is high. Metabolic syndrome suggests a group of disorders including glucose intolerance, central obesity, dyslipidemia (hypertriglyceridemia, elevated no esterified fatty acids (NEFAs), and decreased cholesterol, high-density lipoprotein (HDL), and hypertension. It may manifest in several ways, depending on the combination of the various components of the disorder, and it is well known that it increases the risk of developing cardiovascular disease, type 2 diabetes, and cancer. However, how it begins and how it causally connects the different components between them is still not clear. Different groups of research paid particular attention to one aspect or another. For example, the American Association of Endocrinology does not consider obesity as a factor and emphasizes the importance of the syndrome's insulin resistance. Nevertheless, obesity and the metabolic syndrome do not completely overlap, and now there is clear evidence that there is "benign" obesity. The concentrations of adiponectin plasma in this metabolically healthy obese phenotype are high, in good agreement with the effect of adiponectin overexpression in ob. / ob. mice are resulting in the expansion of fat mass and defense against metabolic comorbidities. The original definition of the World Health Organization considered insulin resistance to be a central feature of metabolic syndrome, whereas the more recent National Cholesterol Education Program (NECP) description: Adult Treatment Panel III (ATP III) applies equal weight to any aspect of the syndrome: glucose sensitivity, obesity, hypertension, and dyslipidemia.

Welsh et al. used a bidirectional Mendelian randomization method to investigate the causal nature of the relationship between adiposity and inflammation and concluded that higher levels of adiposity from fat mass and obesity-associated gene and melanocortin receptor 4 single nucleotide polymorphisms resulted in higher levels of C-reactive protein (CRP), with no proof of reverse trends. While this interesting finding needs to be validated and applied to other inflammatory markers, it helps in the chronic inflammation associated with metabolic syndrome that we focus on adipose tissue. Whatever their roots, whether the key initiator is obese or not, the chronic low-grade inflammatory disorder that accompanies the metabolic syndrome has been implicated in both the development of the syndrome and its related pathophysiological effects as a major player. In good agreement with this understanding of events, weight loss in obese patients is regularly tested to correlate with a reduction in inflammation biomarkers accompanied by an increase in metabolic parameters, that is, insulin sensitivity.

6.7. Cardiovascular Disease

Throughout recent years, common inflammation markers (such as CRP, IL-6, and TNF-alpha) have been identified in the prediction of coronary events; in this regard, CRP is the most important marker for cardiovascular disease.

Danger factors: Circulating high levels of inflammatory markers such as CRP, TNF-alpha, and IL-6 is associated with increased risk of developing cardiovascular disease; even certain acute-phase reactants may also lead to pathogenesis. Even though the recurrent elevation of CRP levels is in a mild degree, it is an independent predictor of future cardiovascular events even within a normal value range. Stratified CRP levels of < 1, 1-3 and > 3 mg / L result in low, moderate and high risk of future cardiovascular events. Previous to this, multiple studies have found a significant correlation between CRP and cardiovascular risk. This finding was first observed over 50 years ago, where heightened CRP level after myocardial infarction was identified as a predictor of poor prognoses. Later, the European Concerted Research on Thrombosis and Disorders Angina Pectoris Study Group indicated that CRP concentrations were higher in patients with coronary events than in those without such events. The Cholesterol and Repeated Events Trial also showed that elevated CRP levels are associated with a significant risk of coronary events following myocardial infarction. Inflammation has been gradually becoming a strong indicator of potential cardiovascular events.

Additionally, hs-CRP is a better proxy for cardiovascular disease than other acute-phase reactants, cytokines, and molecules of soluble adhesion. Therefore, backed by a large number of observational studies and meta-analysis, CRP is considered a mediator of cardiovascular disease, regardless of age, smoking, rates of cholesterol, blood pressure, and diabetes, among other standard risk factors assessed in the clinical setup. Therefore, CRP is one of the most well-documented risk factors for the onset of cardiovascular disease care. Some interventional research using the Mediterranean diet and others marked by increased consumption of mustard or soya oil, fruits, vegetables, nuts, and whole grains decreased cardiovascular disease levels with important anti-inflammatory effects. Several observational and interventional work has shown that intakes of omega-3 and omega-6 fatty acids and alpha-linolenic acid contribute to lower cardiovascular disease incidence and lower inflammatory marker concentrations. Moreover, multiple studies have shown that statin therapy is associated with reduced inflammation and decreased risk of cardiovascular disease.

6.8. Diabetes

Researches have shown that subclinical systemic inflammation predicts diabetes development, as measured by elevated levels of CRP and IL-6[142–149]. It can actually interfere with insulin signaling by inducing proteins that bind to the insulin receptor. A growing body of evidence in this regard supports the hypothesis that chronic systemic inflammation in peripheral tissues contributes to a decrease in insulin sensitivity.

Risk factors: Several studies on healthy subjects have confirmed the relationship between insulin resistance and elevated levels of CRP and cytokines IL-6 and TNF-alpha. Moreover, it has been shown that low-grade chronic inflammation in individuals with impaired glucose tolerance is related to glucose metabolic disturbances.

It has been documented that TNF-alpha is overexpressed in the adipose and muscle tissues of obese and insulin-resistant nondiabetic subjects, an overexpression positively associated with insulin resistance. Ironically, the circulating TNF-alpha levels in type 2 diabetes are higher than in IFG / IGT. In addition, several cross-sectional studies demonstrated an improvement in CRP levels in patients with diabetes, and an increase in CRP, IL-6, and TNF-alpha in IGT subjects.

In addition, certain kinases such as protein kinase C isoforms, I kappa B Kinase-β, and c-jun-terminal kinase have been elevated in obesity, and these kinases have been involved in altering insulin signaling by promoting serine phosphorylation of insulin receptor substrates along with suppression of this substratum's tyrosine phosphorylation. Additionally, various

78

studies have shown that excess nutrient and obesity are associated with elevated levels of free fatty acids that can cause both peripheral tissue insulin resistance and innate immunity activation.

Furthermore, cut-point values for determining the risk of developing the disease are difficult to set, as intermediate CRP values are at moderate risk for metabolic disturbances. Nonetheless, patients with diabetes and CRP values > 3 mg / L were reported to have a 51 % higher risk of all-cause mortality and a 44 % higher risk of cardiovascular mortality relative to those with diabetes and CRP <3 mg / L of comparable age and sex, regardless of classical risk factors such as lipids, blood pressure, and glycemia.

Healing therapy: In the clinical area, there are numerous therapeutic choices, such as genetic, biochemical, and pharmacological targeting of inflammatory signaling pathways enhancing insulin action, which is a central problem in type 2 pathophysiology of diabetes. Existing evidence for inhibiting the cascade of multiple inflammatory kinases in animal models enhances the action of insulin. Thiazolidinediones pharmacological therapies demonstrated anti-inflammatory effects that inhibited both the role of adipocytes and macrophages in obesity and type 2 diabetes. Numerous clinical studies have shown improvements in beta-cell function, and response to insulin decreases in glucose levels, the use of anti-inflammatory drugs to treat type 2 diabetes, and even pre-diabetes. In addition, other studies in patients with type 2 diabetes taking statins have shown a beneficial and additive effect on inflammation levels, which could be an alternative therapy for this condition; however, recommendations for clinical practice should be discussed about the proper use of statin therapy, as specific studies have documented contradictory results with respect to the disease.

The cause of inflammation during obesity and the underlying molecular mechanisms causing its prevalence are not yet fully understood, but pro-inflammatory cytokines do play a central role. In obesity, inflammatory cytokines show higher circulating concentrations than in lean beings, and they are suspected of playing a role in insulin resistance induction. Adipose tissue in obesity is the main source of pro-inflammatory cytokines; it is released mainly by the infiltration of macrophages, while adipocytes play a role. Obesity stems from a number of risk factors, including increased energy consumption and insufficient exercise. Patients with obesity, such as cardiovascular disease, diabetes, metabolic syndrome, and NAFLD, have many difficulties predicting, among others, the risk of future cardiovascular events and death. Different mechanisms have been suggested, including antioxidant, anti-inflammatory, fiber intake, and antiestrogenic processes, to clarify the protective role of certain dietary components, in particular Mediterranean dietary components, which could be a significant change in the clinical lifestyle to prevent the development of metabolic diseases.

6.9. Athletes and Inflammation and the role of antioxidants

The endurance athletes and coaches also pose these questions: How do we preserve good health and improve performance? Are there dietary strategies that promote good health during periods of intense exercise and competitive planning? Are diet or antioxidant supplement intakes effective, and if so, which approach is best? Scientists and clinicians are also interested in these issues, and a concerted effort has been made to identify the clinical and performance effects of supplementation and the physiological mechanisms underlying it in laboratory and field-based research.

This study explores some of the important aspects of the antioxidant supplementation of endurance athletes, including increased free radical production and subsequent oxidative stress caused by high loads of endurance training, the effect of endurance training and oxidative stress on immune function, the influence of improved antioxidant status on performance, recovery and adaptation factors, two special factors

6.10. Oxidative Stress and Endurance Training

Endurance athletes like those who participate in individual running, cycling, swimming, and triathlon events undergo multiple hours of aerobic exercise training each week. Endurance training focuses on the use of oxygen in the skeletal muscle in order to provide the energy needed for such activities. This training's oxidative nature can stimulate the production of highly reactive free radicals, and antioxidant defenses are needed to protect cells from free radical harm. This potential for destroying cells is known as oxidative stress and may result in the inflammatory response of the immune system to protect host tissues.

There is significant evidence that high-intensity or prolonged endurance-training loads promote increased free radical development and oxidative stress (Watson et al., 2005). Preparation for endurance yields increased production of reactive oxygen species (ROS) (Powers and Jackson 2008) and of reactive nitrogen species (Reid 2001; Powers and Jackson 2008).

The most widely formed ROS in cells are superoxide and nitric oxide (Powers, Jackson 2008). While oxidative stress can induce an inflammatory response, free radicals can also play a significant physiological role in training adaptations. There was considerable debate about whether excessive antioxidant intake would reduce training-related adaptations (Gross et al. 2011). It may be difficult for many endurance athletes to strike the right balance between pro-oxidants and antioxidants (Atalay et al. 2006; McGinley et al. 2009).

Regular physical activity can also reduce oxidative stress and inflammation, and improve immune function (McTiernan 2008; Shanely et al. 2011). The length, intensity, and difficulty of exercise activity affects this relationship. Although high-intensity endurance training can increase the activity of antioxidant enzymes and decrease markers for exercise-induced oxidative stress (Miyazaki et al. 2001), extremely high training loads are associated with an acute reduction in antioxidant ability and an increase in oxidative stress markers (Neubauer et al. 2008). This impact has also been shown in athletes who participate in ultra-endurance events, including ultramarathons and ironman triathlons (Knez et al. 2007; Neubauer et al. 2008; Turner et al. 2011). Basically, athletes need to change exercise loads to prevent an increased risk of fatigue, illness, or injury.

Importance of antioxidants Anti-oxidants protect the body against oxidative stress and therefore prevent damage to a wide range of cellular structures, including lipids, proteins, and DNA (Martin 2008). In general, antioxidants are graded as either endogenous or exogenous in the body. The main endogenous antioxidants are superoxide dismutase, catalase, and glutathione peroxidase enzymes, and glutathione. Exogenous antioxidants come from the diet and include, but are not limited to, vitamin E (tocopherols and tocotrienols), vitamin C (ascorbic acid), coenzyme q10 and carotenoids. These compounds have different biological effects, some by converting free radicals into less reactive substances, others by binding supply-lowering proteins, and others by acting as free radical scavengers (Knez et al. 2007; Powers and Jackson 2008).

In preparation for the competition, endurance training places major acute and chronic demands on physiological, metabolic, and energetic processes. Meeting nutrient demands can be a challenge for athletes. Competition for key nutrients during prolonged exercise training between the active and immune systems is one reason that some athletes are at elevated risk of illness. Athletes, who want to add or increase their intake of antioxidants via either dietary sources or supplements, have many choices. Antioxidant supplements are increasingly being marketed in general and sporting communities, with numerous claims about enhanced energy quality, faster recovery from exercise, and improved cardiovascular and immune health. Supplement use is common among endurance athletes enrolled in college athletes in the USA with daily consumption levels of up to 90 percent (Frioland et al. 2004).

6.11. Endurance exercise and symptoms of respiratory illness

One of the most common reasons an elite athlete has to pose for medical examination (Robinson and Milne 2002) is upper respiratory symptoms, and a proven link exists between the training load and the risk of respiratory disease (Walsh et al. 2011). Many athletes suffer from recurrent upper respiratory episodes. Such symptoms are consistent with an inflammatory response and have until recently been thought to be the result of upper respiratory infection. Nonetheless, this isn't always true, and the etiology of the airway inflammation in endurance athletes is varied (Spence et al. 2007), including infection, acute inflammation, allergy, and poorly managed asthma.

While moderate amounts of exercise are usually safe, high volumes of training can increase the risk of respiratory symptoms relative to inactive or moderately active individuals (Nieman 1994). High-intensity, high-volume, or both endurance training events that trigger temporary changes in immune cell function, may be responsible for a period of increased vulnerability to infection that is clinically significant. The risk of upper respiratory tract disease is assumed to be highest during periods of overreaching or overtraining, and around competition. A period of increased vulnerability, the so-called' window of immunosuppression' after exercise, is based on data that shows that immune disturbances can last up to 72 h after competition or a hard training session (Nieman 2007).

Acute neutrophilia and lymphopenia, a decline in natural killer cell activity and T-cell function, a decline in salivary IgA, and higher in pro-inflammatory cytokines and chemokines can be summarized as follows briefly (Nieman 2007). Some changes in the cellular and soluble elements of the immune system have been well established. For these immune responses, it is believed that catecholamines, adrenaline, blood flow, body temperature, and dehydration are among the biological regulators (Nieman 2007).

The underlying infectious cause of athletes suffering from upper respiratory symptoms is not always well established. The belief that inflammation, which is not associated with infection, plays a significant role, is well known in many clinical presentations. In a study investigating the etiology of upper respiratory symptoms in elite athletes, bacterial infections accounted for only 5 percent of the presentations (Reid et al. 2004), with other inflammatory factors responsible for 30–40 percent of upper respiratory symptoms. In support of this finding, viral etiology was identified to the general population in just 30 percent of athletes with the disease with different pathogens (Spence et al. 2007). Epstein–Barr virus reactivation has been shown to be responsible for 22 percent of athletes with chronic symptoms (Reid et al. 2004). Asthma, asthma, and untreated non-breathing diseases and autoimmune disease are some causes of upper respiratory disease in athletes (Spence et al., 2007).

As a result of severe mechanical stress on the airways, exhaustion, and exposure to agents (pollutants, irritants, allergens) able to cause airway damage, athletes may also be at increased risk for airway injury. Such effects are due in large part to the huge and common air motions associated with endurance training. Oxidative stress has been identified as a major factor in contaminant-induced bronchospasm, but only a few studies have investigated the impact of these agents on respiratory symptom-induced athletes (Chimenti et al. 2009).

The treatment with antioxidants has the potential to be a valuable dietary technique for athletes at risk of respiratory disease.

Athletes on a high-antioxidant diet, or who consume antioxidant supplements, may have improved immunity from respiratory disease caused by both exercise and pollution; however, research examining such recommendations are lacking. Outside the athletic culture, antioxidants are known to play a role in altering airway inflammation. As compared to a low antioxidant diet, a general community study of asthmatic individuals examined the role of a high antioxidant diet (Wood et al. 2012). In this study, the low antioxidant diet resulted in a deterioration of two commonly used indicators of asthma intensity (percentage of forced expiratory volume predicted in one second, and percentage of forced vital capability predicted, increased concentration of the inflammatory marker C-reactive protein in serum, and decreased the time for acute asthma exacerbation compared to high antioxidant levels Given the evidence that inflammation involves a significant number of upper respiratory symptoms experienced by athletes, and a significant reduction in airway inflammation is associated with increased intake of dietary antioxidants in non-athletic subjects, a comparable protection can be given to athletes by supplementing the diet with antioxidant-rich foods. More experimental work in athletic groups is required to test this hypothesis.

6.12. Effects of Inflammation on performance, recovery, and adaptation

There is only limited evidence of the correlation of decreased sports performance with respiratory inflammation and infections. A decline for results has been associated with an episode of respiratory symptoms before international competitions for elite swimmers (Pyne et al. 2005). Endurance events such as a marathon, ironman race, or triathlon can cause muscle damage and an acute inflammatory response – though there is also a related rise in anti-inflammatory cytokines (Suzuki et al. 2006). The balance between inflammatory and anti-inflammatory effects depends on a number of factors. The increase in ROS produced in the skeletal muscle during physical activity depends on the intensity and duration of the task being performed and also on the capacity to antioxidant. Though low levels of ROS activity tend to improve (in vitro) contractility, high levels can impair function. Several studies have tried to reduce the adverse effects of exercise through the use of antioxidant-rich supplements. A drop in creatinine kinase and urinary 8-hydroxy-guanosine has been reported following pre-season supplementation with a combination of antioxidants and amino acids in college soccer players (Arent et al., 2010). Although the players showed no benefit from the results, this could mean a potential gain from recovery. Acute supplementation of trained cyclists with a pine bark extract, Pycnogenol, increased fatigue time, total oxygen consumption, and performance 4 hours before an exercise trial (Bentley et al. 2012). Another research that supports the theory of increased antioxidant potential has investigated the effect of supplementing cherry juice on maximum voluntary contractions compared to an energy-matched knee extension placebo (Bowtell et al., 2010). Cherry juice supplementation significantly improved the recovery of isometric strength following exercise as compared with the placebo. While this study is not specific to endurance athletes, the results support the idea that increased availability of antioxidants can delay fatigue time and promote muscle recovery that may improve performance (Bowtell et al., 2010). Before prolonged exercise (2.5 hours of running), blueberry intake resulted in higher NK cell counts and higher anti-inflammatory cytokine concentrations relative to a control group (McAnulty et al., 2011).

Quercetin is one of the few antioxidant supplements that have been tested and shown a strong performance benefit in a number of studies; however, the trials were mostly conducted using untrained subjects. A significant rise in untrained subjects was noticed in a 12-minute treadmill test running results study

(Nieman et al. 2010). In another study, the mean oxygen consumption and cycle time to exhaustion were increased after seven days of quercetin supplementation as compared to placebo (Davis et al. 2010), again in untrained subjects. It is uncertain that highly trained athletes would see that benefit.

One topic of much discussion in sports nutrition is whether the use of supplements can affect normal physiological processes. Many researchers argue that antioxidant supplementation can interfere with the cellular signaling role of ROS and thus prevent adaptations required to improve performance (Gross et al. 2011). The alternative view is that dietary supplements simply increase natural antioxidant capabilities, given the very high demands associated with endurance training and overestimate the fear of physiological interference. In order to overcome this dispute, further studies are needed.

6.13. Dietary vs. Supplement sources of antioxidants

A common problem for athletes is whether they need enough nutritional supplements or antioxidant intakes from usual dietary sources. Inconclusive evidence exists that treatment with anyone antioxidant is sufficient to prevent oxidative damage from exercise-related free radicals or to prevent exercise-related immune disorders or respiratory inflammation (Nieman 2008).

There's a lack of evidence to address this question in athletes. Nevertheless, the view has arisen in people with asthma that whole foods or multi-formulation supplements containing more than one antioxidant may be more effective in enhancing antioxidant capacity (Wood et al., 2012).

A Mediterranean diet allows the general population to fend off oxidative stress. The ATTICA study, a comprehensive epidemiological review of 3000 residents of urban and rural areas surrounding Greece's Athens, identified important linkages between adherence to the Mediterranean diet and health benefits (Kontogianni et al. 2012). Higher overall antioxidant ability and lower rates of low-density oxidized lipoprotein (LDL) cholesterol have been associated with good adherence to this diet. It is believed that reducing LDL-cholesterol accounts for its protective effect on cardiovascular health. This study further proved a link between the Mediterranean diet and decreases in inflammation and coagulation markers.

While a high antioxidant diet is associated with reduced inflammation of the airways and severity measures in patients with asthma and chronic airway disease (Wood et al. 2012), there is some concern about the effectiveness and even protection of supplementation with one single high-dose antioxidant. For example, experiments in the form of α-tocopherol combined with isolated vitamin E have increased oxidative stress markers, somewhat counterintuitive, over placebo during the Triathlon World Championships (Nieman et al., 2004).

A variety of dietary antioxidant supplements including quercetin, blueberries, and even cherry juice (Nieman et al. 2007, 2010; Bowtell et al. 2010; Davis et al. 2010; McAnulty et al. 2011) demonstrated the potential for improvement in exercise outcomes. Multi-nutrient supplementation may be a safer choice compared to very high doses of individual antioxidants, or nutrients that provide improved antioxidant protection, with lower potential harm risks (Atalay et al. 2006). A diet rich in natural antioxidants is best recommended, with ample amounts of a variety of fruits and vegetables.

6.14. Ultra-endurance events and altitude training

Ultra-endurance events are an area of endurance exercise and sport which warrants special consideration for dietary antioxidant supplementation. These events attract significant numbers of competitors from both non-elite amateurs and professional endurance athletes. The most well-known of these extreme events is the ironman triathlon with a 4-km swim, 180-

km bike, and a complete 42-km marathon (Knez et al., 2007; Turner et al. 2011). Research investigating the effect of full and half-ironman triathlons on oxidative stress markers found that at rest, the ultra-endurance athletes had lower levels compared with relatively inactive controls (Knez et al. 2007), but post-competition elevations showed a significant inflammatory response. These athletes had relatively higher levels of erythrocyte antioxidant enzymes at rest but decreased in post-race enzymes that suggest a lack of antioxidant defense mechanisms. Oxidative stress levels may remain elevated following a sustained physical activity for many days. In an Ironman triathlon race, Neubauer et al. (2008) observed improvements in a variety of oxidative stress markers; after the event, these markers had taken five days to return to baseline (Neubauer et al. 2008).

The athletes taking antioxidant supplements may have higher levels of oxidative stress than age-matched, relatively inactive control subjects after half or full iron man triathlon competitions (Knez et al. 2007). Similarly, vitamin E (α-tocopherol) supplementation, two months before an ironman case, caused higher elevations of oxidative stress in post-race markers than placebo (Nieman et al. 2004). Another research investigating the impact of ultra-marathon swimming on oxidative stress (Kabasakalis et al. 2011) found no significant difference between pre-and post-race markers of oxidative stress, possibly due to the low-intensity nature of this activity compared to that studied in other sports which are at a higher average percentage of peak VO2. Another study investigating oxidative stress factors in response to swimmers ' training activities found that pre-and post-training flavonoid-based juice supplements did not reduce oxidative stress after exercise despite higher rates of oxidative stress compared with inactive controls (Knab et al. 2013).

The impact of altitude training requires special attention since altitude exposure can increase the production of oxidative stress irrespective of the duration or amount of exercise (Bakonyi and Radak 2004; Pialoux et al. 2009a, b). Therefore, it seems possible that during this period of heightened oxidative stress, increasing the supply of antioxidants would improve health, and possibly exercise. Studies were conducted using the altitude exposure method called' sleep high, exercise low.' Endurance training with intermittent resting hypoxia resulted in lower rates of antioxidant plasma resting without hypoxic exposure, with little change in the control group (Pialoux et al. 2009b). The restorative hypoxia community also reported a greater rise in post-training oxidative stress markers. Training with the added hypoxia tends to cause an increase in the production of free radicals, which depletes the body's antioxidant ability. The increased intake of antioxidants should help maintain antioxidant levels during this period. The loss in the hypoxia population did not return to baseline levels after two weeks of recovery (Pialoux et al. 2009a), indicating a more sustained impact on antioxidant concentrations. Other studies reported only a small difference in markers of oxidative stress in the supplemented population after two weeks of moderate-intensity exercise at high altitude (Subudhi et al. 2004). Amid prolonged submaximal cycling (55 percent VO2 max), the concentration of oxidative stress factors did not improve in this study. The increased oxidative stress caused by altitude exposure can play a significant role in adaptation, and dampening this effect with antioxidant supplementation can potentially impede adaptation.

Antioxidants can reduce the possible oxidative stress produced by high volume and intensity of endurance training. However, it is not absolutely clear whether increased oxidative stress triggered by training is, in fact, detrimental to the athlete. Further research is warranted by the degree to which an increase in free radical production during high training loads influences the signaling required for adaptations to training. When solving these issues, athletes should seek advice from their health care practitioner(s) on antioxidant supplements that should assess individual requirements in terms of underlying health, nutritional diets, and training loads.

There's some evidence that increased dietary antioxidants change the course of the disease in diseases with an inflammatory etiology. Diets that increase fruit and/or vegetable intake (and therefore high in dietary antioxidants) are likely to have a number of unknown beneficial biological activities that are not measurable or observable. Further research is needed to decide whether nutritional approaches that help the disability groups in the general community, such as those with asthma, are transferred directly to hard-working but otherwise healthy endurance sportsmen.

Mixed antioxidant-rich diets can be safer than antioxidant supplementation and may offer greater benefits. Higher antioxidant intakes may help maintain a normal antioxidant / antioxidant balance. Supplementation with antioxidants can benefit endurance athletes undertaking extremely high levels of training, either living and/or exercising at moderate to high altitudes or participating in ultra-endurance competitions.

6.15. Athlete's guide to fighting inflammation

Exercising intensively triggers the release of substances known as free radicals. Free radicals can cause damage to the cells, loss of muscle function, and cause an inflammatory response. Eating antioxidant-rich foods and omega-3s helps protect the cell membranes from damage caused by these free radicals. Both nutrients contribute to the development and healing of damaged tissue and can help improve short-and long-term recovery from intense exercise.

6.16. Foods that fight inflammation

Vegetables-Rich in vitamins & antioxidants such as vitamins A, C, flavonoids, and carotenoids, vegetables are no brainer to help fight inflammation. Many of the richest sources include bell peppers, tomatoes, green leafy vegetables such as, but are not limited to, kale, spinach, and collard greens, beets, mushrooms (also high in vitamin D), broccoli, and sweet potatoes.

Berries–Research has shown that, before and after intense exercise, athletes who eat berries experience decreased inflammation and oxidant stress. The berries contain many antioxidants, including anthocyanins, vitamin C, and resveratrol. Add a variety to your diet, including blueberries, strawberries, goji berries, raspberries, and blackberries.5 Egg yolks–yolks are rich in vitamins including vitamins A, C, lutein, and zeaxanthin. While egg white omelets are often mistaken for being a "healthier" option, actually, the yolks you want are the ones. On all of those foods, you miss eating only the whites.

Whole grains–Because of their high fiber content, whole grains such as quinoa, brown rice, and oats can help protect against inflammation. Spices-Some spices, such as ginger or turmeric, contain anti-inflammatory compounds. Apply certain herbs to your dishes along with garlic or add a pinch to your smoothies.

Seeds-Seeds like flax and chia are high in fiber and omega-3 fatty acids. Baseball players-keep eating those sunflower seeds in the dugout! They're high in vitamin E and essential fatty acids.

Nuts–Rich in good antioxidants like vitamin E and anti-inflammatory fatty acids like omega-3, nuts should be a staple in your response to inflammation. Find a variety that includes almonds, walnuts, cashews, and pistachios.

Fatty fish–Fatty fish such as salmon, mackerel, herring, sardines, and albacore tuna are all high in omega-3 fatty acids. Although I always recommend food always but if you don't eat enough of these omega-3 rich foods in your diet, then you need to take an additional supplement, make sure you use a safe and approved drug. Search for the "NSF Certified for Sport" tag and ask a dietitian before beginning any new supplement.

The Tart Cherry Juice-Cherries are extremely rich in antioxidants. This concentrated cherry juice has been shown to reduce inflammation.

Citrus fruits-Citrus fruits are rich in protein, flavonoids, and vitamin C and can help combat inflammation and strengthen the immune system. Apply more citrus fruits like bananas, lemons, limes, and grapefruits to your diet.

Avocados-These "fruits" have anti-inflammatory effects, high in monounsaturated fats, vitamin E & C, and fiber. They are an excellent replacement for highly saturated fat spreads, such as mayonnaise or butter, on bread and sandwiches.

6.17. Foods to avoid

Refined starches such as pasta, white bread, and rice rapidly break down into sugar during the digestive process, which in turn may lead to inflammation, especially in high quantities. Inflammation can also lead to excessive amounts of added sugar such as glucose, fructose, molasses, a concentrate of fruit juice, high syrup of fructose corn, and syrup, to name a few. Consider raising the amount of fried, canned food that you consume, including cakes, crackers, cookies, and cereals. If sugar and flour are the first two ingredients, then pass it on and look for a better alternative.

In addition, **high intakes of trans and saturated fats may cause inflammation.** Monitor the intake of red meat and processed meat since they occur to be higher in saturated fat. Hydrogenated and "Partially Hydrogenated" (Trans Fat) are the most common in fried foods, snack foods, and sweets such as pastries, cookies, candies, and crackers. Read the ingredients, Mark. If the ingredient "partially hydrogenated" is listed, skip it.

Alcohol in moderation, mainly red wine due to its antioxidant content, can indeed be a good thing. But, going well beyond this "moderation" stage (i.e., no more than one women's drink, two men's drinks) could actually do more harm than good to your body.

6.18. Meal planning tips

Incorporating the foodstuffs described above can help to combat inflammation. Here are a few simple ideas/recipes which will help you put it into a meal plan.

Breakfast- Make a 2-egg omelet with peppers, onions, spinach, and mushrooms, or put it all together at the Casserole Market Breakfast from this farmer. Have a large bowl of fried berries. For athletes requiring additional calories, provide a side of oats with walnuts on top.

Lunch & Dinners- Take advantage of a grilled or broiled fish filet like salmon, lean protein like a chicken breast, or plant-based protein like quinoa bed lentils or brown rice. Finish with a heaping cup of green vegetables like broccoli or kale, season the platter with garlic, ginger or turmeric. To add some extra calories and healthy fats, chop up half an avocado and sprinkle the sesame or pumpkin seeds on top. Then render this Burrito Bowl with a Recipe.

Snacks- Enjoy fresh fruits and veggies like bananas, onions, carrots, or cucumbers eaten with a blended nut. Then dip apple slices into peanut butter than almond butter. Have a slice of whole-grain bread spread on top with almond butter, berries and flax seeds or mix in a smoothie with a variety of fruits and vegetables. Enjoy a glass of cherry juice, or make it into a smoothie-like your milk.

6.19. Reducing inflammation and Promoting recovery in athletes

Do you know inflammation is a normal part of the workout? Inflammation naturally occurs after a hard workout to help athletes heal muscles, and athletes can improve and adapt to more challenging workouts as the training continues.

Sleep well! Nonetheless, too much inflammation can become a problem that results from too many hard workouts with insufficient attention to recovery nutrition, adequate sleep, and unhealthy diets, and can have a negative impact on sports performance and impair immunity, which can lead to days off from practice or competition. Many athletes can turn to non-steroidal anti-inflammatory drugs (NSAIDs), such as ibuprofen, to decrease inflammation and reduce pain, but these drugs have been linked with stomach damage, and may potentially impede training adaptations that help athletes recover fast.

Soreness is part of daily training, but rather than popping up NSAIDs, with the following healthy diet and rest strategies put more focus on recovery and inflammation-fighting: make sleep a priority! The muscles rest and regenerate during sleep, and poor sleep can increase inflammation in the body. Increasing sleep and/or napping to a minimum of 8 hours can improve performance, mood, decrease tiredness, and improve reaction times and concentration.

Remove refined carbohydrates such as white rice and white bread, soda, French fries, and other processed foods such as crispy fried chicken, chips,pizza, and frozen fruit cakes, which may cause inflammation.

Add extra products to your plate by eating more antioxidant-containing fruits and vegetables, and phytochemicals that combat inflammation. Include anti-inflammatory foods in your daily diet, especially during periods of heavy training, such as tart cherry juice, turmeric, and fish oil.

Boost your consumption of healthy fats by snacking on walnuts, almonds, peanuts, flax seeds, using olive oil as a dressing on salads, and eating fatty fish like salmon and tuna for your protein for few meals a week to reduce inflammation.

Reducing or avoiding alcohol – over-consumption of alcohol can cause inflammation and disrupt sleep, which can be detrimental to long-term health together.

Eat enough calories to compensate for your physical activity and ensure the right amount of carbohydrates, protein, and healthy fats (macronutrients) is ingested. Not eating enough calories will increase the stress hormones, leaving athletes unable to fight off inflammation and heal properly after a hard workout.

Taking the holidays off! Rest days following intense workouts are an integral part of a training routine that helps athletes recover and make the next practice or match even better. Athletes who are running down, like they can't recover from their last practice/competition or see improvements in their performance, should speak to their coach about their training and take a look at their choice of diet and lifestyle to see where they can improve.

A sports dietitian will work with your workout schedule and current diet to help you achieve your goals for success this season by developing a nutrition plan that will help you perform better and get stronger through this season.

Chapter 7: Dietary Factors that have an impact on Inflammation Related to obesity

Diet is a key factor in controlling immune responses. There is considerable evidence that malnutrition is contributing to immune-suppression because of a vulnerability to infection. On the other hand, over-nutrition leads to immune-activities, due to a susceptibility to an inflammatory disorder. Hence an optimal diet is needed for a healthy immune balance.

7.1. Carbohydrate

Carbohydrates are a significant source of dietary energy and can be measured using the GI and GL values. GI is a food classification based on their postprandial reaction to blood glucose, and a carbohydrate quality calculation. GL is a metric measuring both the amount and strength of the dietary carbohydrates. Large cross-sectional studies have demonstrated an association of GI / GL and inflammatory cytokines in the diet. In the Women's Health Research (n=13.187, > 45 years of age), the large quintiles of dietary GL and GI were significantly related to high blood levels of C-reactive protein (CRP). Similarly, in Dutch research (n=974, 42-87 years old), the highest quintile of dietary GI and GL was positively correlated with blood levels of CRP ($p<0.05$). In addition, the Nurse Health Survey (n=902, aged 30-55) and the follow-up survey of health professionals (n=532, aged 40-75)[39] found that a high GI or GL diet was significantly associated with low plasma adiponectin levels ($p<0.05$). The high levels of CRP and low levels of adiponectin in the blood are characterized as a low-grade inflammatory disorder associated with obesity. Ironically, inflammatory cytokine (CRP, TNF-α, and IL-6) randomized clinical trials did not exhibit a relationship between a high GI or GL diet. Nevertheless, 30 percent of the energy restriction in the high GL showed a decrease in serum CRP concentration in healthy overweight adults (n=34, 24-42 years old). Several detailed observational research found a positive correlation between a high GI/GL diet and inflammatory markers; however, the intervention studies could not convincingly support this association.

7.2. Dietary Fat

A high-fat diet induces excessive body fat accumulation, which affects the immune system. A variety of different fatty acids, including polyunsaturated (PUFA), saturated, and trans-fatty acids, have been examined for their effects on inflammatory conditions. Joffe et al. recently reviewed the effects of dietary fatty acids on gene expression and on the development of TNFα andIL-6.

PUFA omega-6 (n-6) PUFA and omega-3 (n-3) PUFA families are precursors of eicosanoids which play an important role in the immune response. Cross-sectional studies have identified the n-3 PUFA (eicosatetraenoic acid[EPA] and docosahexaenoic acid[DHA]) anti-inflammatory activity. The Nurses' Health Study I (n=727, aged 43-69) and the Attica Survey (n=3,042, aged 18-89) found that the consumption of n-3 fatty acids or fish is inverted to inflammatory biomarkers (CRP, IL-6, and TNF-α) (p<0.05). Interventional research (n=30, mean age 60 years) also reported that supplementation of fish oil (14 g / d of fish oil for five weeks) in healthy postmenopausal women decreased blood CRP andIL-6 levels.

Trans and saturated FA Observational and interventional research indicate a clear correlation between trans-or saturated FA and immune response. According to the Nurses ' Health Research I Cohort (n=730, 43-69 years of age), the highest quintile of trans-FAs intake was associated with high levels of CRP andIL-6 compared with the lowest quintile. In a randomized crossover trial (n=50), replacing trans-FAs (8%) with a high-fat diet (39% of fat) essentially increased blood levels of CRP and IL-6 (p<0.05). Likewise, replacing trans-FAs (< 7%) with a standard diet (30% of fat) increased the levels of

109

IL-6 (as well as the levels of TNF-α but not CRP) in subjects with mild hypercholesterolemia.

7.3. Vegetable, fruits, and other nutrients

Numerous cross-sectional studies and some observational studies have documented an inverse correlation between high rates of vegetable and fruit consumption, either in combination or alone, and CRP. The Boston Puerto Rican Health research (n=1,159, 45-75 years of age) also found that variable fruit intake associated inversely with blood CRP levels. In addition, Salas-Salvadó et al. (n=772, 55-80 years of age) and Freese et al. (n=77, 19-52 years of age) didn't show any link with inflammatory markers (adiponectin, CRP, IL-6, intercellular adhesion molecule-1[ICAM-1], vascular cell adherence molecule-1[VCAM-1]) between a vegetable and fruit-rich diet. Morand et al. (n=24, mean age 56) found that a single fruit supplement (500 mL of orange juice/d over four weeks) did not affect the levels of CRP, IL-6, ICAM-1, and VCAM-1.

Other Nutrients: Several vitamins and minerals have been shown to have beneficial effects on oxidative stress and immune responses. The association of vitamins and minerals with inflammatory marker levels (CRP, TNF-α, and IL-6) has been consistently demonstrated by cross-sectional and interventional research.

Vitamin A: Overweight or obese participants frequently reported lower plasma carotenoids due to the high proportion of carotenoids found as lipid-soluble compounds in adipose tissue. The Women's Health Study (n=2,895, aged around 45 years) reported higher plasma α-and β-carotene concentrations associated with low plasma CRP rates.

Vitamin C, in general, has beneficial effects on immunity. Aasheim et al. demonstrated that low plasma vitamin C levels were substantially associated with elevated levels of CRP in subjects with severe obesity (62 men and 106 women aged 19-59). Block et al. (n=216) supplemented vitamin C (515 mg / d over eight weeks) in stable smokers. They observed that supplementation with vitamin C significantly reduced levels of blood CRP (24 percent, $p<0.05$). In comparison, Fumeron et al.[58] (n=42, aged 18-80) confirmed that vitamin C supplementation (750 mg / d for eight weeks) did not change blood levels of CRP.

Magnesium (Mg): Mg intake was inverted to dose-dependent levels of CRP, IL-6, and TNF-α-R2 in the Women's Health Study (n=3,713, 50-79 years of age), following adjustment for multiple variables, including dietary fiber, fat, meat, and vegetables. Guerrero-Romero and Rodríguez-Morán showed that low serum Mg levels were independently linked to elevated CRP concentration in non-diabetic, non-hypertensive obese subjects (n=371).

Flavonoids: A subclass of polyphenolic biological compounds, flavonoids are present in plant-derived vegetables, nuts, spices, chocolate, tea, and red wine. Several intervention studies have demonstrated strong antioxidant properties of flavonoids; however, their inflammatory and immune-regulatory effects are less clear. The Nurses ' Health Study (n=2,115, 43-70 years of age) found that low levels of pro-inflammatory biomarkers(IL-18 andsVCAM-1) were correlated with a diet rich in flavonoids (flavones, flavanones, and full flavonoids). The U.S. recently The Department of Agriculture (USDA, 2006) (n=8,335, around 19 years old) confirmed that high dietary intake of flavonoids was inversely associated with plasma concentration of CRP ($p<0.05$). A randomized, parallel controlled study (n=120, 40-74 years of age) found that the supplementation of bilberry juice (300 mL / d for three weeks) decreased plasma levels of pro-inflammatory cytokines (TNF-α, IL-6, and-8, with no changes in CRP). Karlsen et al. recently reported that the use of bilberry

112

juice (330 mL / d for four weeks) significantly reduced plasma levels of pro-inflammatory cytokines (TNF-α, IL-6, and IL-15) and CRP in CVD-risk subjects (n=62, 34-68 years of age). By contrast, a double-blind, placebo-controlled crossover study (n=14, 35-53 years old) found that marine buckthorn flavanol extract supplementation for four weeks did not reduce CRP levels (p<0.05)

7.4. Phytoestrogens, probiotics, and prebiotics

Phytoestrogens are plant origin compounds found in a wide variety of foods, beans, nuts, and grains. It's assumed that phytoestrogens have anti-inflammatory properties. A diet of naturally isoflavone-enriched pasta, aglycones (33 mg / d), decreased plasma CRP concentrations significantly in a randomized, controlled study. When the subjects were changed back to a traditional diet (n=62, mean age 58.2 years), plasma CRP levels returned to baseline. Meanwhile, in a study of healthy postmenopausal women, the supplementation of soy isoflavone (genistein at 54 or 40 mg / d) for six months did not affect rates of CRP (n=30, 50-60 years of age, and n=80, mean age 49.5 years). Similarly, in a study of obese postmenopausal women, soy isoflavone supplementation for six months had no impact on plasma CRP concentration (n=50, mean age 58).

There are studies that the supplementation of phytoestrogen has beneficial effects on inflammatory markers, but the results are contradictory.

Probiotics are living micro-organisms that provide a health benefit to their host. Orally ingested probiotic bacteria can modulate the immune system; however, different probiotic strains may have different immune-modulatory effects. In a randomized, double-blind, placebo-controlled trial, in healthy subjects (n=30, 23-43 years of age), the combination of Lactobacillus gasseri and Lactobacillus coryniformis with Staphylococcus thermophilus had no effect on serum TNF-α or IL-12 concentrations. Comparisons with L were made by Kekkonen et al. Bifidobacterium ssp animalis. Rhamnosus lactis Bb12, and propionibacterium freudenreichii ssp. Shermanii JS during three weeks in healthy subjects (n=81, ages 23-58). There was no effect on serum levels of TNF-α, IL-6, IL-10or IFN-ÿ but a reduced level of CRP in the L. Group of rhamnosus supplementation. Although it has been shown that probiotics have beneficial effects on inflammatory markers, further studies are needed to arrive at the definitive results.

Prebiotics are non-digestible elements of food that provide a health benefit to the host associated with the regulation of microbiota in the gut. The IL-6 mRNA expression decreased by oligofructose, a common form of prebiotics, supplementation (8 g / d for three weeks) in the elderly (n=19, mean 85 years of age). By contrast, oligofructose supplementation (1.95-3.9 g / d for 12 weeks) had no effect on IL-6 or TNF-α plasma levels in poorly nourished elderly subjects (mean age 70 years). Although a convincing correlation between a prebiotic supplementation and inflammatory markers has been shown by a few observational studies, drawing this beneficial association is currently premature.

7.5. 1,200 Calorie Anti-inflammatory diet plan for weight loss

The anti-inflammatory diet is about consuming more of the foods that help to reduce inflammation in the body while reducing the foods that tend to increase inflammation, thereby helping to fight inflammatory conditions. The diet includes many colorful fruits and vegetables, high-fiber legumes and whole grains, healthy fats (such as those found in salmon, nuts and olive oil) and antioxidant-rich herbs, spices and tea, thus minimizing processed foods made with unhealthy trans fats, refined carbohydrates (such as white flour and added sugar), and too much sodium.

In this healthy 1200-calorie meal plan, they put together the principles of anti-inflammatory eating to offer a week of tasty, wholesome meals and snacks, plus meal-prep tips to set you up for a good week ahead to achieve weight loss.

As inflammation can be caused by many other factors in addition to food, such as low rates of exercise, stress, and lack of sleep, it can also help prevent inflammation by incorporating healthy lifestyle habits into your daily routine. Combine this balanced meal plan with daily physical exercise (aimed at moderate intensity for 2 1/2 hours a week), stress-relieving exercises (such as yoga, meditation or something that works best for you), and a good night's sleep every night (at least 7 hours a night), to get the most anti-inflammatory benefits. Whether you're working actively to minimize inflammation or just searching for a balanced diet plan, this 7-day anti-inflammatory meal plan will help.

Meal prep for a week

At the beginning of the week, a little meal prep will set you up for healthy-eating success.

Prepare the Vegan Superfood Buddha Bowls for Days 2, 3, 4, and 5 to have lunch. Refrigerate the bowls and separate dressing for up to 4 days. Avoid until you are ready to eat, adding avocado to avoid browning.

Make the Tahini Dip with Turmeric-Ginger to have snacks throughout the week.

Day 1:

Foods that contain high omega-3 fatty acids, such as salmon, sardines, and albacore tuna, have been shown to reduce levels of inflammation. Try to include at least two portions of 3-ounce fish rich in omega-3 fatty acids each week.

Breakfast (287 calories): 1 serving overnight Blueberry-Banana Oats, 1 cup of green tea

Lunch (325 calories): 1 serving Green Salad with Edamame & Beets

Snack (117 calories): 2 Tbsp. Turmeric ginger tahini dip. 1 carrot. Cut that into sticks

Dinner (442 calories): 1 serving Walnut-Rosemary Crusted Salmon, 1 serving Roasted Squash & Apples with Dried Cherries

Daily Totals: 1,202 calories, 57 g of protein, 131 g of carbohydrate, 30 g of fiber, 54 g of fat, 1,520 mg of sodium.

Day 2:

Anti-inflammatory bonus: An antioxidant, vitamin C has anti-inflammatory properties because it helps to decrease dangerous free radical cells that can cause inflammation. Studies prove that people with diets high in vitamin C have lower levels of the C-reactive protein inflammatory marker as well as a lower risk of inflammatory diseases, such as gout and heart disease. Today's Raspberry-Kefir Power Smoothie provides 45 percent of Vitamin C's recommended daily value!

Breakfast (249 calories): 1 portion Raspberry-Kefir Power Smoothie A.M.

Snack (28 calories): 1/3 cup of blueberries

Lunch (381 calories): 1 serving Vegan Superfood Buddha Bowl P.M.

Snack (9 calories): 1/2 cup of sliced cucumber flavored with a pinch of salt and pepper each.

Dinner (393 calories): 1 serving Indian-Spiced Cauliflower & Chickpea Salad, 5 ounces of water (drained) Bottom tuna salad.

Evening snack (156 calories): 1 ounce of dark chocolate

Daily total: 1,215 calories, 70 g of protein, 143 g of carbohydrate, 35 g of fiber, 47 g of fat, 1.054 mg of sodium

Day 3:

Anti-inflammatory bonus: Anthocyanins are strong antioxidant compounds found in dark blue fruits and vegetables, red and purple, as well as red wine. Research suggests that anthocyanins parts a role in decreasing signs of inflammation, which can reduce cancer risk and heart disease. Keep frozen berries on hand to give your morning smoothies or oatmeal an anti-inflammatory boost, so you can get the benefits even when they're not in season!

Breakfast (263 calories): 1 cup of low-fat plain Greek yogurt 1 1/2 (Blueberries 1/4 cup sliced walnuts 1 cup green tea Top walnuts and blueberries yogurt.

Snack (42 calories): 2/3 cup raspberries

Lunch (381 calories): 1 portion Vegan Superfood Buddha Bowl P.M.

Snack (117 calories): 2 Tbsp Turmeric ginger tahini.

Dinner (409 calories): 1 portion Superfood Chopped Salad with Salmon & Creamy Garlic Dressing

Daily Totals: 1,212 calories 77 g of protein, 97 g of carbohydrate, 28 g of fiber, 63 g of fat, 813 mg of sodium.

Day 4:

Anti-inflammatory bonus: moderate intake of dark chocolate and cacao will reduce inflammatory markers and improve heart health. Cocoa is rich in flavanol quercetin, a potent antioxidant that protects our cells, and a major component of the anti-inflammatory diet is dark chocolate. Incorporate the darkest chocolate one 1-ounce square a day that you will find to maximize benefits.

Breakfast (222 calories): 1 portion Cocoa-Chia Pudding with Raspberries

A.M. Snack (109 calories): Half cup low-fat Greek yogurt with 1/4 cup of blueberries

Lunch (381 calories): 1 portion Vegan Superfood Buddha Bowl

P.M. Snack (9 calories): 1/2 cup sliced cucumber Pinch of salt Pinch of pepper Dinner (472 calories) 1 serving Stuffed Sweet Potato with Hummus Dressing

Daily Total: 1,191 calories, 56 g protein, 168 g carbohydrate, 49 g fiber, 39 g fat, 1,100 mg sodium

Day 5:

Anti-inflammatory bonus: Probiotics such as those present in kimchi, yogurt, kefir, and kombucha help support healthy intestines. Research shows a healthy gut is enhancing our immune systems, helping to maintain a healthy weight, and reducing inflammation. Always make sure to include prebiotics, which are indigestible plant fibers found in foods such as garlic, onions, and whole grains, which help to provide fuel for good bacteria to improve our gut health.

Breakfast (249 calories): Raspberry-Kefir Power Smoothie

A.M. Snack (2 calories): 1 cup of green tea

Lunch (381 calories): 1 Vegan Superfood Buddha Bowl

P.M. Snack (58 calories): 1 tablespoon Turmeric-Ginger Tahini Dip with 3/4 cup sliced cucumber

Dinner (414 calories): 1 portion Korean Steak, Kimchi & Cauliflower Rice Bowl Evening

Snack (120 calories): 5 ounces of red wine

Daily Totals: 1,224 calories, 57 g of protein, 112 g of carbohydrates, 28 g of sugar, 53 g of fat, 1,067 mg of sodium.

Day 6:

Anti-inflammatory bonus: Any form of arthritis, an inflammatory joint condition, which is often treated with a mixture of an anti-inflammatory diet and prescription medication, affects more than 20 percent of U.S. adults. The best anti-inflammatory diet for arthritis involves a lot of magnesium studies, which indicates that it reduces inflammation and helps to maintain joint cartilage. Many Americans don't get enough magnesium, so make sure to include plenty of nuts, legumes, whole grains, and seeds to ensure adequate intake.

Breakfast (249 calories): 1 serving Raspberry-Kefir Power Smoothie

A.M. Snack (157 calories): 12 walnut halves

Lunch (325 calories): 1 serving Green Salad with Edamame & Beets

P.M. Snack (78 calories): 1/2 ounce of dark chocolate

Dinner (401 calories): 1 serving Hummus-Crusted Chicken 1 serving Blistered Broccoli with Garlic and Chiles Meal-Prep Tip: Cook and save the extra chicken for lunch. You will require two cups of cooked chicken, chopped.

Daily Total: 1,209 calories, 73 g of protein, 94 g of carbohydrate, 28 g of fruit, 63 g of fat, 1,245 mg of sodium.

Day 7:

Anti-inflammatory bonus: A diet rich in fiber would have a lower glycemic index, a measure of how our blood sugars are affected by food. Fiber is slowly digested, which keeps us full and enhances the regulation of blood sugar. Additional bonus-eating food is lower on the glycemic index that helps lower levels of C-reactive protein, which is a marker for inflammation. A balanced anti-inflammatory diet provides a total of 28 grams of fiber every day.

Breakfast (292 calories): 1 serving Cocoa-Chia Pudding with Raspberries 1 Turmeric Latte

A.M. Snack (42 calories): 1/2 cup of blueberries

Lunch (350 calories): 1 serving Avocado Egg Salad Sandwiches

P.M. Snack (116 calories): 15 unsalted almonds

Dinner (448 calories): 1 serving single-pot Garlicky Shrimp & Spinach 1 cup of cooked quinoa

Daily Totals: 1,209 calories, 62 g of protein, 128 g of carbohydrate, 32 g of fiber, 55 g fat, 1,362 mg sodium.

Chapter 8: The Anti-Inflammatory Lifestyle

Inflammation is one of the natural ways the body defends itself. This involves multiple chemical reactions that help fight off infections, increase blood flow to places where healing is needed, and create pain as a sign that something is wrong with the body. Unfortunately, as any process in the body, one can possess too much of a good thing.

Inflammation is sometimes equivalent to an acid. There is no doubt that fire keeps us dry, protected, and covered in limited quantities, but it can be dangerous when there is too much fire, or when fire gets out of control. But that doesn't have to be high for damage to cause a fire. It is now evident that low-grade chronic or recurrent inflammation, which is below the level of pain, can contribute to many chronic problems of health and can become a disease itself. This low-grade inflammation can prevent proper tissue healing and can also start killing healthy cells in the lungs, muscles, joints, and other parts of the body.

Too much inflammation is associated with a range of medical conditions. Some of these include:

• Alzheimer's disease

• Asthma

• Obesity

- Chronic obstructive lung disease (emphysema and bronchitis)

- Chronic pain

- Type 2 diabetes

- Heart disease

- Inflammatory intestinal disease (Crohn's disease or ulcerative colitis)

- Stroke

- Body-attacked disorders such as rheumatoid arthritis, lupus, or scleroderma.

The most famous test is to check your blood for the amount of C-reactive protein (hsCRP).

How to prevent or reduce excessive inflammation: In order to reduce inflammation, people often take medicines. Drugs such as ibuprofen and aspirin can change the body's chemical reactions but are not without side effects. Research has shown that lifestyle choices can also minimize inflammation; our choices can affect the degree to which we have inflammation within our bodies. Adapting to a healthy diet as well as other healthy lifestyle habits can have a dramatic effect on inflammatory levels.

8.1. What is an Anti-inflammatory lifestyle?

The anti-inflammatory lifestyle includes the following features:

- Consuming anti-inflammatory food
- No smoking
- Reducing alcohol intake
- Adequate exercise
- Getting enough sound sleep
- Stress management
- Weight management

8.2. Eating to reduce inflammation

Everything we eat can affect inflammation, and certain foods are more likely to reduce the effects of pain and other illnesses. Approximate 60 percent of chronic diseases could be avoided by a healthy diet, including many of the health problems listed above.

2 Consuming the right foods can not only mitigate the onset of inflammation in the first place but can also help to reduce and resolve chronic inflammations.

Anti-inflammatory way of eating: Reducing inflammation is not one-size-fits-all. A number of people would do it differently. The traditional Mediterranean diet, influenced by some

Mediterranean basin nations, is one of the most researched examples of an anti-inflammatory way of eating.

Those who regularly follow a Mediterranean-like diet have significantly lower inflammatory levels compared to other less balanced approaches to food.

The Mediterranean diet protects against many chronic conditions, including cardiovascular disease, type 2 diabetes mellitus, Alzheimer's and Parkinson's disease, and some cancers.

The Mediterranean diet is just 1 example of a traditional diet and seems to be the best-researched traditional diet in the world. Most traditional diets are healthier than current popular diets, as they concentrate on eating organic, unprocessed foods, shared with family and friends. The specificities of the Mediterranean Diet that vary from study to study, but these are often common elements.

Usually (though not exclusively), the **Mediterranean diet** is a plant-based diet, rich in fresh fruits and vegetables, whole grain cereals, and legumes. It advocates nuts, seeds, and olive oil as fat sources and needs moderate intakes of fish and shellfish, eggs, white meat, and fermented dairy products (cheese and yogurt), and relatively small amounts of sweets and red and processed meats. It is possible that the diet as a whole, rather than individual contents, leads to good results. The various components work together to reduce the inflammation and bring about beneficial effects in the body.

Several primary aspects of the Mediterranean diet include:

- Relatively high fat intake (30-50 percent of total daily calories) o Usually from monounsaturated fatty acids (mainly olive oil) o Saturated fats make up less than 8 percent of calories.
- Heavy fruit and vegetable intake
- Low fiber consumption (32 g / day)
- High in easily digested carbohydrates (i.e., low glycemic load). For more details, please see Managing Better Health Dietary Carbohydrates. The Mediterranean diet is just 1 example of a typical diet pattern. In general, traditional diet patterns are safe, anti-inflammatory patterns because they do not contain processed foods.

8.3. Consuming more anti-inflammatory food

Eat a vibrant, well-balanced diet with lots of vegetables and fruit: Diets high in fruits and vegetables that provide essential antioxidants and phytochemicals with good anti-inflammatory nutrients; some beneficial plant substances, called phytochemicals, include brightly colored fruits and vegetables, usually green, orange, black, red, and purple. Most of these compounds have antioxidant properties that can assist in minimizing inflammation. Studies show a diet high in fruits and vegetables is beneficial. Fruit and vegetables: The more you cook, the better you eat. A good target of a variety of vegetables and fruits, including dark green, brown, yellow, red, and legumes (beans and peas), is at least 4 1/2 cup-equivalents per day. Of sweet, "soft" vegetables like lettuce, and raw spinach, one cup counts as 1/2 cup-equivalent. One-half cup counts as an average of 1/2 cups for denser vegetables such as peas, green beans, or chopped sweet peppers. Insist on fruit over vegetables. Purple and red berries are particularly full of anti-inflammatory compounds, as are cruciferous vegetables such as broccoli, kale, cabbage, and cauliflower.

Increase the quantity of Omega-3 Fatty Acids: Foods containing long-chain omega-3 fatty acids such as cold-water fish (salmon, sardines, and tuna) are particularly suitable for decreasing inflammation. Typically found in plants, omega-3 fatty acids abundant in fatty fish, eicosapentaenoic acid (EPA) and docosahexaenoic acid (DHA) are more potent anti-inflammatory agents than alpha-linolenic acid (ALA) (2-3 servings of fatty fish such as salmon, mackerel, herring, lake trout, sardines and albacore tuna per week). ALA converts to

EPA and then to DHA, but less than 1 percent of the initial ALA is transformed into the physiologically active EPA and DHA.

For this reason, the ALA-rich flax oil is not as good as EPA and DHA for inflammation. Fish oil contains EPA and DHA (about 18% and 12% respectively) and is a good source of these essential fatty acids. Plant sources of omega-3s usually contain ALA, but now there are vegan supplements derived from algae that contain both EPA and DHA.

Consider adding fresh fish oil to your diet. 1 gm of fish oil contains approximately 0.5-1 gm of total omega-3, so aim 3-4 gm of fish oil per day or 5-4 gm for inflammatory treatments.

Improve intake of olive oil: extra virgin olive oil is an excellent choice when cooking, as it has been shown to be lower in blood pressure, LDL cholesterol, and inflammatory markers.

Pay attention to the oils in popular salad dressings and opt for olive oil where possible. Olive oil contains mainly monounsaturated fatty acids (not omega-3 or -6s) and comes in several grades; "pure' is the most processed,' virgin' has modest processing, and extra virgin olive oil (EVOO) is minimally processed and valued for its presence of many potent beneficial phytochemicals.

Cook well with "Fresh" and "Virgin." It is best not to cook with EVOO as heating it to a moderate temperature will reduce the phytochemical content by around 15 percent-25 percent, but the benefits of monounsaturated fatty acids remain. EVOO may be added after cooking or used for making salad dressings. Canola oil is a better option as a mainly monounsaturated oil, but it does not contain many of the beneficial olive oil phytochemicals, and less research is done to support its anti-inflammatory effects. Certain oils that are relatively high in monounsaturated fatty acids include almond, rice bran, and sesame oils, but they also contain moderate amounts of omega-6s.

Coconut oil: There is growing interest in cooking with coconut oil. Coconut oil is "heart-healthy" or not is currently under discussion. Coconut oil tends to increase more HDL-cholesterol (the "healthy" cholesterol) than LDL-cholesterol (the "poor" cholesterol), thereby leading to a more favorable cholesterol profile compared with butter. Therefore, in the case of traditional diets where coconut oil is consumed daily, this does not appear to cause damage.

This means which it is important to understand the rest of the diet, not just the oil itself. It is suggested that coconut oil, in the context of an unhealthy Western diet, can increase cardiovascular risk. In terms of inflammation, preliminary animal research suggests that extra virgin coconut oil may have anti-inflammatory properties, but there is still a lack of human research.

Using Tea and Other Spices: Spices such as ginger and turmeric contain other important anti-inflammatory compounds to improve those in your diet by drinking teas (green is a strong anti-inflammatory tea) and use those spices in your cooking.

8.4. Avoid inflammatory foods

Avoid trans-fatty acids: Trans fatty acids stimulate inflammation. Items that may contain trans-fats, also referred to as "hydrogenated oils," include margarine, deep-fried foods, and processed foods designed for long shelf life, such as crackers and packaged foods.

Restricted Refined Seed Vegetable Oils: Restrict seed oils (soybeans, corn, sunflower, grapes, cotton seeds, and wheat germ oils) and processed foods high in omega-6 fatty acids, and select sources of monounsaturated fatty acids, such as canola and olive oils, while increasing the intake of omega-3-rich foods (such as fatty cold water); The seed oils given above are not necessarily harmful in limited amounts.

It's just that they're a lot of in the western diet.

The history story on omega-6 fatty acids Omega-6 fatty acids is abundant in the traditional western diet. These are found in high concentration in the conventional seed oils mentioned above, and hence in many processed foods (crackers, chips, fast foods). What effect omega 6 fatty acids have on inflammation and on chronic health conditions remains unclear. Recent research has suggested that there is too much interaction between these dietary fatty acids and body proinflammatory pathways. Nonetheless, more recent research suggests that omega-6 fatty acids may not directly increase inflammation, and may actually act in an anti-inflammatory manner, depending on other factors.

What is evident, however, is that omega-3 fatty acids, like those from cold-water fish, have anti-inflammatory, and thus beneficial health effects.

What can you think about it?

The evidence suggests that human beings evolved between omega-6 and omega-3 on a diet with an essential fatty acid ratio of about 1:1. The current western diets are in the range of around 10-25:1.

Yet ancient humans ate a lot fewer omega-6 than conventional fatty acids in America. Since seed oils are so widely used in most processed foods, the best way to reduce your omega-6 intake is by reducing processed foods in your diet.

All fatty acids omega-3 and-6 are essential nutrients in your diet, so you need some omega-6s, but you should limit them. Hence, focus on increasing the dietary omega-3s and reducing the dietary omega-6s while maintaining all essential dietary fats.

Reduce Saturated Fat Consumption: Recent evidence continues to indicate that food with high dietary saturated fat consumption in the context of an unhealthy Western diet is associated with low but increased risk of cardiovascular disease and low but increased rates of inflammation, especially for overweight and obese people.

Nonetheless, when reducing saturated fat, the emphasis on poly-and monounsaturated fats and particularly omega-3 fatty acids, rather than carbohydrates, is crucial. In the context of the whole diet the intake of the aforementioned anti-inflammatory foods leads to a positive synergistic effect.

• Regular dairy consumption Full-fat and non-fermented dairy products may have a small effect on increased inflammation, but overall, dairy products do not appear to increase inflammation. Moreover, fermented dairy products such as yogurt and Kiefer have a neutral or even positive effect on cardiovascular risk and inflammation. Consumption of dairy products, especially yogurt in regular amounts, may be learned. To be sure to minimize sugar intake, choose basic, unsweetened varieties.

Regulate the intake of red meat: Those consuming the most overall red meat remain at the highest risk of diabetes, cardiovascular disease, and multiple cancers. Recent evidence, however, suggests that the main culprit may be the processed red meat, such as hot dogs, sausages, and lunch meats.

Red meat is one of the good sources of protein, iron, and other micronutrients, but it can be a good substitute for poultry, eggs, and dairy as well as vegetable proteins (legumes) and grains. Pick unprocessed grass-fed sources that may have more desirable fatty-acid profiles if you eat red meat, pick lean cuttings, and trim visible fat. The World Cancer Research Fund recommends 12 to 18 ounces of red meat per week (three 6 oz servings or six 3 oz servings), cooked weight; 3 oz is about the size of a card deck. Avoid processed foods like bacon, salami, hot dogs, and sausages.

Giving Charring up: Food Charring is related to inflammation.

Reduce Blood Sugar: The body easily breaks down foods high in refined carbohydrates such as white flour, rice, bread, and refined sugar into simple sugars that are rapidly absorbed and can cause large spikes in the hormone insulin that promote inflammation. Better to limit or avoid such foods.

Eat low-GL: eat low-GL foods and meal plans (see Managing Better Health Carbohydrates).

Those include complex carbohydrates (such as unprocessed whole grains, starchy vegetables, and fruits), foods high in protein, fat, and fiber that help balance blood sugar and reduce the inflammatory effects of insulin. As complex carbohydrates are consumed in conjunction with high-fiber foods and healthy oils, carbohydrate degradation is delayed, and the overall glycemic load is that.

Consume More Fiber: Diets high in fiber aim to reduce inflammation.

Fiber helps slow the absorption of carbohydrates, helps to control blood sugar levels, and also helps to keep you full longer. Mechanisms by which fiber minimizes inflammation are not fully understood, but fiber promotes fat recycling in the body, and also attracts "clean" bacteria in the intestines that have a positive effect on inflammatory pathways. Complete, fiber-rich foods often contain several essential phytochemicals with anti-inflammatory properties.

The fiber target is 30 grams a day, or more. Get used to reading packaged food nutrition labels to help you find more fiber options for the products. Nevertheless, fiber is better derived from whole foods. Total fiber intake can be difficult to keep track of, but if you eat a healthy diet pattern like the Mediterranean diet, you usually get plenty of fiber. See the tips below for some safe ways to increase your fiber intake.

Ensure adequate Magnesium: (Mg) intake deficiency is associated with increased inflammation. Due to poor nutrition, Mg is under-consumed in the US, and it is estimated that 60 percent of Americans do not get enough. Dark green vegetables are an affluent source of Mg as well as legumes, nuts, seeds, and whole grains. The recommended dietary allowance (RDA) for Mg for females and males over age is 320 and 420 mg / d, respectively. It does not appear that consumption beyond that point gives any further benefit. One cup of spinach or Swiss chard contains about 150 mg; 1/4 C of pumpkin seed contains 190 mg; 1 Cup of black beans, 3/4 C of quinoa, and 1/4 C of cashew or sunflower seed contains about 120 mg, respectively.

Be patient: It takes some time for the anti-inflammatory eating to work. Try them for at least six weeks or longer. Eventually, it must become a natural way of eating in order to keep you safe over the long term.

Fiber Tips Change your carbohydrate sources to full-food carbohydrate sources such as starchy vegetables, legumes, whole grains, and fruits, keeping your glycemic load small.

One-half cup starchy vegetables (beets, corn, green peas, parsnips, winter squash, sweet potatoes, and pumpkin) contain around 2-4 grams of fiber. One medium apple contains 4 to 5 grams of fiber, and about 3.5 grams of fiber originates from a medium orange. Carbohydrates shape around a quarter of your plate.

The legumes: Eating at least one serving (1/2 cup) of legumes (beans and peas) every day can go a long way for gaining your target of fiber. A 1/2 cup of cooked lentils, garbanzo or black beans contains 6 to 9 grams of fiber. All beans are a good source of obtaining fiber and create a variety in your diet, add it to soups, and use pureed beans as dips and spreads (think hummus!). Start slow to prevent excessive gas and to bloat; the body eventually adapts.

Use whole grains over refined grains. Entire grains are treated minimally so that the whole grain remains intact. Whole grains contain oats, brown rice, quinoa, millet, barley, buckwheat, bulgur wheat, amaranth. 1/2 cup includes 2-4 grams of fiber

• Include and eat vegetables in each meal. One study indicated that when people ate a salad before the main meal, they consumed 23% more vegetables than those eating salad at mealtime, increased their fiber intake and lowered their calorie intake

8.5. Tips to an anti-inflammatory lifestyle

Being healthy exercise has been shown to reduce inflammation, and people who get regular physical activity have lower levels of inflammation. Guidelines for physical activity include:

A cumulative goal of 150 minutes (30 minutes 5 days a week) of moderate aerobic physical activity such as tennis or walking, or 75 minutes (1 hour and 15 minutes a week) of intense physical activity.

Muscle-reinforcing workouts (such as weight training or resistance bands) of medium to high intensity on two days or more a week.

Get Enough Quality Sleep: Sound Sleep is one of the most important things people need to keep their minds and their bodies healthy. The Centers for Disease Control suggests that approximately 35 percent of US adults do not get the optimum 7 hours of sleep a night. People who do not get enough sleep or who have frequent interruptions or poor quality sleep are more likely to have more inflammation and also health problems such as type 2 diabetes and weight gain.

Manage stress: Stress exists in many ways, such as physical (hazard threat), mental (job or financial stress), and emotional (social rejection, isolation, or relationship stress).
Stress is a part of life and may change during life. If stress is overwhelming or if there is moderate ongoing stress that is not relieved, the body could lose its ability to respond healthily, resulting in increased inflammation that could harm our health. It can build the ability to manage stress. All of the above techniques— eating a healthy diet, getting active, and getting enough sleep — improve the ability of the body to deal with life stresses. Certain approaches like mind-body strategies like mind-based stress reduction (MBSR), progressive muscle relaxation (PMR), biofeedback, breathing exercises, yoga, and tai-chi can be useful.

Weight management: Inflammatory equilibrium in the body is caused by several factors. Some evidence indicates maintaining a healthy weight may be important for inflammation management. People who are obese, or who have excess abdominal weight, have a higher risk of inflammation than others. In particular, those located in the abdominal area, fat cells (known as adipocytes), develop and secrete compounds that can lead to inflammation. Fortunately, even a small weight loss of 10% of body weight can help to reduce inflammation. Aim of a healthy diet like a Mediterranean diet or an anti-inflammatory diet.

Description: Each of those lifestyle factors can aid in reducing inflammation. Bite off a convenient bit, and change one at a time. This will help improve and retain the ability to make changes. Trying to find a balance in your life, handling stress in a healthy way, being part of a community, spending time outside, doing exercise, sleeping well, and, most importantly, spending time with people you love is just as vital as eating food. You must feed yourself as a whole—mind, body, heart, and spirit.

Note: The recommendations here are detailed suggestions for a dietary plan, which can help to reduce inflammation.

Individuals may have particular sensitivities to the food, which may contribute to inflammation.

Chapter 9: The inflammatory diet to avoid in order to cure various inflammatory diseases

The elimination diet is the eating program that omits a food or group of foods that are believed to cause an adverse food reaction, often referred to as "food intolerance." By avoiding certain foods for a period of time, and then re-introducing them during a "challenge" period, you will identify the foods that cause symptoms or make them worse. We also think of food reactions as a sudden allergic reaction, like a person getting an anaphylactic reaction to eating peanuts and swelling their throats.

However, there are several other ways our bodies react to foods that might not be so immediate and may or may not be correlated with an immune response. Food intolerances can be induced by various natural compounds found in foods (natural sugars or proteins) or by common food additives (such as natural and artificial colors, preservatives, antioxidants, and taste enhancers) that can trigger reactions via different mechanisms in the organism. The precise mechanisms involved in the different food reactions are still being discussed, and many studies may be unsuccessful in identifying the suspected culprit(s). Clinical experience has shown that a diet on elimination is one of the best resources for identifying food culprits and is very healthy as long as a variety of foods are still eaten containing all the nutrients needed.

9.1. Symptoms

Symptoms of food intolerance can vary widely. These can involve the stomach and abdominal swelling, headaches, hives, itching, and even vague signs of being unwell, such as flu and pains, extreme tiredness, or concentration problems. It is also known that certain foods and food groups intensify symptoms in people with specific illnesses, such as autoimmune disorders, migraines, irritable bowel syndrome, gastroesophageal reflux (GERD), and others. Symptoms and severity are special to the person. They are affected by different compounds in the food, a person's level of sensitivity, and how much those foods are consumed. By consuming the same food on a regular basis or eating different foods together or regularly with the same ingredient, the body may reach a threshold or tipping point where symptoms begin to develop.

Natural Food Substances: Only "healthy" foods contain a number of different chemicals that occur naturally, and for some people can be a concern. Substances similar in various foods, such as salicylates, amines, and glutamate, may cause different people symptoms. Providing information about the different categories of natural substances that may cause symptoms is beyond the scope of this handout, but this can be addressed with a practitioner who is comfortable working with removal diets (not all practitioners are).

Human variability: Because people are genetically unique, and each of us has various eating patterns, increasing human needs to focus on diets for elimination. The most successful way of finding out which foods can contribute to the symptoms is to remove the most offensive food or many foods and substances all at once. A healthcare practitioner can recommend that a particular plan be followed based on symptoms, typical dietary choices, and food cravings.

9.2. The Elimination Diet Steps

The Elimination Diet has four key steps:

Step 1
Planning Consult with your health care provider to find out which foods may cause problems. You will be asked to keep a

diet log for a week, list the foods you consume, and keep track of the symptoms you have for the entire day. See the final page of this handout for a Food Diary Poster, which you can use.

A few main questions to ask yourself are helpful:

• Which foods do I eat the most often?

• What foods do I want?

• Which foods do I eat to "feel better"?

• Which foods would I have trouble giving up?

Sometimes these seem to be the most important things to look for and not eat. Make a list of issues of potential foods.

Depending on how many suspicious food culprits are avoided, the extent of the elimination diet can differ. It is possible to follow three different "levels" of food exclusion based on potential food culprits and the probability of adhering to the diet. The three levels are listed below in the Eliminating Diet Strategies section on page 6. First of all, it is helpful to consider choosing the approach that is the least restrictive in order to optimize successful adherence to the restrictions. Nevertheless, more rigorous methods are more effective in identifying cases that involve multiple culprits against food.

Are You Ready?

It is important to consider before beginning a diet on elimination, whether it is a good time to undergo these

148

potentially large changes in diet. Do you have any planned stressful events or lifetime journeys? Do you have the money, will, and ability to create new cooking lists and menus?

Are you supported by family and friends for eating at home, at college, at restaurants, and other events? It will be important to remove the foods on your list entirely for 2-4 weeks, so if you somehow accidentally eat one of the foods, you'll have to start again. If you succeed the first time, it's going to be faster and easier.

Step 2

Make a list of foods to avoid depending on your planning, and be sure to avoid potential "hidden products" (see table 3).

Begin the elimination diet, and maintain the elimination diet for two to four weeks without exception.

Do not eat as a whole or as ingredients the foods excluded from other foods. For instance, if you avoid all dairy products, you need to check the whey, casein, and lactose labels to avoid them as well. The step requires much discipline. Food labels should be very cautious. Be particularly careful when eating out, as you have less control over what's going into your food. If you make some mistake and eat something on the list, then you should start over again.

Most people notice their symptoms may get worse in the first week, especially during the first few days, before they begin to get better. If your symptoms escalate or become serious over a day or two, contact your health care practitioner.

Step 3

If your signs have not improved in two weeks, live for up to 4 weeks. If your symptoms have not better by the end of 4 weeks, leave the diet and start retrying this process with another combination of foods.

• You should be free of symptoms for at least five days before the challenges of your food start. If your symptoms have improved, start with the discarded foods of your body, "challenging" one meal at a time. Use the Food Diary to keep a record of your symptoms in writing at the end of this paper.

• Add new food to body check every three days. It takes three days to make sure that the symptoms will have time to return if they so wish. You are recommended to eat a small amount on Day 1of re-introduction, have about twice that amount on Day 2, and then an even larger portion on Day 3. See Table 2 for an example calendar. Notice that certain foodstuffs are essential.

It is suitable in small quantities but not in larger quantities. In recognizing these foods, keeping a careful dietary log may be of great help.

• Testing with the purest available form of food is essential. For example, use a pure wheat cereal, which includes wheat only to be tested for wheat. A non-dairy milk alternative such as rice or other milk may be used as long as that milk is not on the "stop" list. Check the milk and cheese in separate occasions. Similar cheeses may or may not have different sensitivities, so it's best to check them separately. Usually, yogurt, cottage cheese, and butter do not have to be tested separately. For chickens, the whites and yolks are separately tested using hard-boiled eggs.

• The food issues should be tackled in the most systematic way possible. Many food elements, such as the proteins casein and whey, and dairy sugar lactose, can be routinely separated by careful challenge planning. Try working with a professional health care provider who can assist you in planning your plan when you suspect a particular component of a food may be a culprit. However, when you exclude an entire food group, it may only be acceptable to challenge the category of one or several different foods, not every single item.

• Delete the item from the diet as soon as the symptom returns, take a note of it, and place it on the "allergic" list in the food diary. If you are unsure of responding to a meal, remove it from your diet and recheck it within 4-5 days. If a food does not cause symptoms during a challenge, it is unlikely to be a problematic food and may eventually be added back to your diet.

Nonetheless, don't put the food back during this phase of the program until you've completed the diet and the food challenges. In other words, go back from that diet before it is over to fight for all the foods you have taken out.

Step 4

By eating them, your health care provider can help you plan a way to avoid your symptoms, based on your results. Some things to keep in mind: • This is not a perfect test. It can be extremely difficult to tell for sure that if a particular food is the source. The findings could be interfered with by many other factors (such as a stressful day at work). Try to keep food as consistent as possible when taking the diet.

• Many people have more than one problem with food.
• Make sure you get enough daily care and change your diet over the long run. For example, if you give up dairy, you will need to replace your calcium from other sources such as green leafy vegetables.
• You may need to try multiple different elimination diets before identifying the food problem.
• Many people tolerate this diet well, but if you exercise with the diet many times in an attempt to narrow down the food culprits, the list of allowed foods maybe even smaller. If this

happens and you find yourself becoming more intolerant to food or losing enjoyment, please contact a healthcare professional to advise.

• You may have access to certain foods that you are susceptible to on an infrequent or rotational basis. If required, consult with a health care professional to learn how to plan for this.

9.3. Elimination of Inflammation Diet Strategies

Level 1: Simple *(Modified) removal of meat (or dairy and gluten-free)* - This is the lowest-resistance diet. There are two ways to do that. The food, party, or substance in question is focused on the symptoms and alleged culprits.

1. If one item is missing, one food group or one food additive. See Table 1 for the most common culprits in food. This is the easiest diet to adopt, but if symptoms are triggered by more than one food or food group, then this diet may not be helpful. Avoiding only the dairy food category would be perfect for the alleged allergy to lactose. Alternatively, lactase is the enzyme that digests disaccharide lactose and can be administered as an over-the-counter medication. When the lack of lactose causes symptoms to disappear, on occasion, milk can still be enjoyed with the help of lactase.

2. Instead, it removes the two most common culprits in the food group (dairy and wheat). The most common types of food protein that can cause intolerance are the milk protein and wheat gluten in the cow.

• Exclude all dairy products, including milk, butter, sausage, cottage cheese, fruit, cookies, ice cream, and frozen yogurt.

• Exclude gluten, including wheat, spelt, Kamut, oats (allowed to be gluten-free), rye, barley, or malt. This is the principal component of the diet. Substitute products with brown rice, millet, buckwheat, quinoa, gluten-free flour or potato products, tapioca and arrowroot

Level 2: *Low-intensity elimination* - diet In a moderate intensity elimination diet, several foods or classes of foods are removed at once. Ideally, the list of foods excluded is individually modified based on the symptoms and the suspected culprits in the product. For instance, low FODMaP diet may be a good example of symptoms associated with Irritable Bowel Syndrome (IBS) A skilled health care provider can help you identify potential food culprits for your condition or symptoms. Whether complying with the detailed guidelines below and in Table 4 or compiling a custom list. A version of the diet for elimination may be more effective in removing symptoms, as more possible culprits will be removed immediately.

The suggested moderate-intensity elimination diet, in addition to dairy and wheat, excludes meat, all legumes, nuts, several different fruits and vegetables, artificial sweeteners, all animal fats, lots of vegetable fats, chocolate, coffee, tea, soft drinks, and alcohol. This diet will take longer, demanding times to identify the food's culprits. Pay attention to the fact it can be expensive to buy licensed foods.

• Exclude all animal protein; however, where this is not possible or desirable, pork, poultry, and lamb are considered to be a low allergy. Select organic/free-range outlets, wherever possible.

Stop alcohol and caffeine and any papers that may contain these ingredients (including sodas, cold preparations, herbal tinctures).

• Avoid foods containing yeast or foods that promote excessive yeast growth, including processed foods, refined sugars, cheeses, seasonings, peanuts, vinegar, and alcoholic beverages;

• Avoid natural sugars such as chocolate, cookies, and processed foods.

• To drink at least two-quarters of water a day.

Level 3: *The Few-Foods Diet* - This much simpler diet can eat only a small number of foods. This diet should only be followed for a limited period until the food's culprits are detected to ensure no nutritional deficiencies are present.

• This diet is the most restrictive edition and includes only the foods called for in Table 5.

• To help you make the planning process as organized as possible, work with your health care provider;

• This is not a long-term diet consistent with nutrients. In order to ensure proper nutrition, it is necessary to add back foods that do not cause symptoms once the removal time of the diet is over.

9.4. Some Helpful Tips

Looking at food labels, a number of products may be 'disguised.'

If you have an allergy from latex, you can also respond to apple, apricot, avocado, banana, carrot, celery, cherry, chestnut, coconut, fig, shrimp, grape, hazelnut, kiwi, mango, melon, nectarine, papaya, passion fruit, peach, pear, pineapple, plum, potato, rye, shellfish, strawberry, tomato, and wheat.

Conclusion

Inflammation helps the body battle disease and can protect it from injury. In most cases, this is an essential part of the healing process.

However, many people have a medical disorder in which the immune system doesn't function as it should. This failure can lead to permanent or chronically low levels of inflammation. Chronic inflammation occurs in various conditions such as psoriasis, rheumatoid arthritis, and asthma. There's proof that food options can help manage the symptoms. The anti-inflammatory diet favors vegetables and fruit, foods that contain omega-3 fatty acids, whole grains, lean protein, healthy fats, and spices. This prohibits or discourages the use of processed foods, red meats, and alcohol.

The anti-inflammatory diet is a pattern of feeding, rather than a routine. Mediterranean diet and the DASH diet are examples of anti-inflammatory diets.

References

- Anti-inflammatory Diet dishes retrieved from:

https://www.medicalnewstoday.com/articles/322897.php#breakfast

- The elimination diet retrieved from:

https://www.fammed.wisc.edu/files/webfm-uploads/documents/outreach/im/handout_elimination_diet_patient.pdf

- Obesity, inflammation and diet retrieved from:

https://www.ncbi.nlm.nih.gov/pmc/articles/PMC3819692/

- Athlete's guide to fighting elimination retrieved from:

https://www.eleatnutrition.com/blog/inflammation

- The anti-inflammatory lifestyle retrieved from:

https://www.fammed.wisc.edu/files/webfm-uploads/documents/outreach/im/handout_ai_diet_patient.pdf

Lightning Source UK Ltd.
Milton Keynes UK
UKHW021256250721
387668UK00002B/100